THE
PRIVATE
SQUARE

Volume 2: Breasts

TABITHA KATZ

The Private Square
Volume 2: Breasts
All Rights Reserved.
Copyright © 2015 Tabitha Katz

CreateSpace, a DBA of On-Demand Publishing, LLC

ISBN-13: 978-1530791569
ISBN-10: 1530791561

http://www.theprivatesquare.com

PRINTED IN THE UNITED STATES OF AMERICA

Table of Contents

Foreword

The job of an Aesthetic Breast surgeon is to be able to produce larger breasts from small, small breasts from large, symmetric breasts from asymmetric, and in general improve the overall shape and form of the breast mound. Over the past 30 years I have found that this is not as easy as it would appear to be. Why is that? Why is the median perception of breast beauty such a moving target and why does the average size (the mean under the breast size curve) of the mound change from culture to culture and cycle from time to time?

The answer is that in most western cultures, the raison d'être of the breast is more than an organ of caloric nourishment. The ever-changing appreciation of breast form is more a reflection of the changing social and cultural elements that are constantly ebbing and flowing in all populations. In fact, the breast's function as a sexual visual beacon produces more economic output than its primary biological purpose. From fashion designers who highlight feminine body curves to boudoir visual enticements, the power of the breast form is a primary generator of feminine attraction. Its attractive power, however, is not determined by whether the breast form is large or small, whether robotically symmetrical or biologically asymmetric. It is truly the beauty of proportion and curves that elicits a positive sexual response and not the absolute size or form.

The "Breasts," in *The Private Square* series by Ms. Katz, gives all those who doubt that their breasts are within the "mean form and size" of the US population a pleasant surprise in documenting that breasts come in all sizes and shapes, especially when not airbrushed by mercenary publications. Ms. Katz states that the presentation of the breast form is far less important than the woman living inside. As a professional analyst of breast beauty, I wholeheartedly agree…

Andrew M Wolin, MD, FACS
Scottsdale, Arizona

Praise

To my girl. I've sympathized with you over the years as you struggled with the feeling you got the genetic short straw in terms of the size and shape of your breasts. I've felt your pain and triumphs as you grew to realize that your body was just right for you. The adage *"with time comes wisdom"* is true – I know as the years pass you will come to understand there is no such thing as physical perfection. Love yourself and know that to the ones who love you, you are absolutely beautiful.

Thank you for your unwavering support. Thank you for all your help. Know that you are an inspiration to me. I love you.

***To my daughters* and their friends.** You are all just right!

TK

Introduction

As a woman and a mother of three daughters, I have been around many breasts for many decades. Seeing and photographing another 100 pair was not a big deal. What is a big deal is the media/entertainment driven standard for what constitutes nice, even "normal" breasts that has little to do with the way the female body really looks.

In 1970 Judy Blume published her book *Are You There God, It's Me Margaret*. It is about a sixth grade girl coming of age spiritually, emotionally and physically. Breast development, or the lack thereof, was discussed during a meeting of Margaret's girlfriends:

> "If you ever want to get out of those baby bras you
> have to exercise," she told us.
> "What kind of exercise?" Gretchen asked.
> "Like this," Nancy said. She made fists, bent her arms
> at the elbow and moved them back and forth, sticking
> her chest way out. She said, "I must — I must — I
> must increase my bust." She said it over and over. We
> copied her movements and chanted with her. "We
> must — we must — we must increase our bust!"
> "Good," Nancy told us. "Do it thirty-five times a day
> and I promise you'll see the results."

That book became the prepubescent girls' bible. I was 11 years-old when it was published and my breasts had just begun to develop. Even with the proper "exercise," I did not get the kind of breasts I envisioned. For years, I was embarrassed by them. A decade later, after a long-time college friend turned lover proceeded to rhapsodize over my breasts, at 23 years-old I finally accepted my own anatomy.

Many women, but not all, are more comfortable with their breasts and bodies as young adults than they were as teens. For many, body image changes drastically when women decide to become mothers. During pregnancy, breasts take on an entirely different meaning. The physical and functional changes can be dramatic. Post-childbirth, especially post-nursing, breasts are forever altered. Women who formerly were satisfied with the look of their breasts can find themselves feeling quite different. It is not a surprise that the average age for breast implant surgery is 34.

In addition to the changes caused by life events and age, women have to contend with the image propagated by one of the largest advertisers of intimate apparel: Victoria's Secret. Online, on television, in print media and stores, Victoria's Secret models' breasts are everywhere. They are firm, high on the chest, round and voluptuous. Cleavage swells perfectly atop beautiful bras and out of a variety of low necklines. There are no bulges in front of their arm pits (oops, do these models even have arm pits?!?), nor is there any extra fat being squeezed from under the bands or straps. To make us feel better about our breasts, retailers like Victoria's Secret, Frederick's of Hollywood, Bare Necessities, etc., manufacture lingerie in beautiful colors and fabrics, adorning their bras with lace, netting, shimmering metallic thread and more. They size their bras smaller than customary so when you wear their intimate apparel, you are an entire cup size larger – and, don't you know, bigger breasts are more beautiful?

Are these models' bodies even their own? More likely than not, the answer is no because most photos have been retouched to enlarge and reshape breasts and more. So what do "real" women's breasts look like? *Girls Gone Wild* photos on the internet? (Pardon me while I cringe.) Movie stars' breasts on the big screen? (Think there is some pre-screening here?) Very young, select women posing for spreads in *Playboy*, *Penthouse* or other "girly" magazines? Porn stars? No.

Real women's breasts do not follow any prescribed shape or size. Virtually every woman's breasts are to some degree asymmetrical. You, your mother, sisters, daughters, friends and me have breasts that change over time. Female breasts are so much more than just sexual body parts.

Just take a look... and read on.

More Dirty Ditties

Talking about breasts does not have nearly the social stigma that discussing penises does. For women, breasts become a topic of discussion relative to puberty, sexually coming of age, impending motherhood, pre- and post-breastfeeding, before, during and after menopause, and in discussions about breast cancer, health and more. Women discuss their breasts relative to how clothes fit, whether certain exercises cause discomfort, whose are real or fake, etc.

What is not talked about is how we feel about our own breasts. Do we like the way they look or hang? Are they too big, too small, too far apart? How do we feel about the color or size of our nipples (actually called areolae)? What about our breasts' sensitivity or sexual responsiveness?

What do we say to the teenage girl who is taken aback because her breasts do not look like the pictures in lingerie catalogues? How do we respond when a boy is heard laughing with his friends about the girl's breasts he saw that did not look like those in the magazine under his bed? How do we prove to our daughters and sons what real women's breasts look like? Certainly not by opening a *National Geographic* magazine!

Whether you are somewhat unhappy with your breasts or harbor a more serious negativity, these very personal feelings can dampen self-esteem, inhibit intimate relationships or compromise sexual enjoyment. *The Private Square* series attempts to counter personal negativity stemming from societal pressures of measuring up to unrealistic physical perfection by showing you what real people, like you and me, look like - in an honest and unaltered way. Reality, plus a little sense of humor, can truly make us feel better about ourselves.

I took the liberty of modifying *The Private Square* jingle that I first heard from a bunch of middle school 'tween'agers after their state-mandated 7th Grade sex education class:

Boys Verse

Please! Lemme touch you there
Right in your private square
Tatas, patooties and love canal too
Wanna get my hands on you!

Girls Verse

Hey! Don't touch me there
That is my private square
Boobies, tush and my v'jayjay
Unless I say - keep your hands away!

What's In A Name?

The breasts can represent fertility, motherhood and nourishment, sexuality and femininity.

"O! be some other name:
What's in a name?
that which we call a rose
By any other name would smell as sweet"

Romeo and Juliet, Act II. Scene II. William Shakespeare, 1914

The Not-So-Romantic Synonyms For Breasts:

Boobs • Rack • Shimmies • Titties • Boulders
PomPoms • Bosom • Fun Bags • Knockers • TaTas
Jugs • Warheads • Girls • Mammaries • Peaches
Niblets • Bean Bags • Assets • Balcony
Hooters • Globes • Teats • Mosquito Bites
Melons • Fog Lights • Orbs • Bazookas • Tits
Puppies • Apples • ChaChas • Headlights • Lactoids
Bazongas • Twins • Chesticles • Blinkers • Mounds
Honkers • Mammas • BettyBoops • Torpedos
Floaters • Twangers • Woofers • Pointer Sisters
BonBons • Nips • Ear Muffs • Whoppers
Sugar Plums • Dueling Banjos • Cupcakes

Finding Breast Models

Sample Ads

Wanted: women of any age and type (like Dove Everyday Women) as life models for paid professional, anonymous, educational photo shoot. No experience necessary - $40.

Looking for women – any age, size or look to model for educational anatomy project. No faces or full body pictures taken. All photography is anonymous. Payment $40 for individual photo shoot.

Will pay $40 to take anonymous photos of your sexual body parts. No faces or full body pictures taken. Must be 18 or older. Appointments or walk-ins welcome.

Need adults 18 & older for anatomical photography project. The pay is $40 for a 10-minute, anonymous, individual session to take pix of private body parts. Release and receipt must be signed. Studio hours by appointment. Walk-ins are welcome.

Seeking a widely diverse population of women (18 or over) for an educational, anatomical, anonymous photo shoot. Young adults must show proof of age.

Responses

"I'm 21 years old, a French dancer just arrived in USA two months ago and I'm looking forward to meet artists with some projects like yours."

"I'd like to model/be a photography subject for your project tomorrow. I know you said that there will be no posing, but the most releveant experience I have is figure drawing modeling."

"I'm willing to have a photo taken of my private area. Oh– one more thing I'm a black female. Is that ok? I know people have certain preferences for photos and things."

"I am very interested in being in your project! Do you still need body parts? I am a 25 yr old female, M.S. Human Development."

"So the diversity you are looking for are really with the specific body parts, right? Curious."

"I'm an A cup and don't have a very exciting body. I guess I can help out though. Should I shave or wax ahead of time?"

"I have done some freelance art modeling so I'm comfortable posing partially nude or nude. I'm a 20 year-old multiracial female with fully grown-out armpit hair."

"Are you making a book or a research paper or something? I would participating if it's for something helpful to others."

"I'm not your skinny girl – I am a big boned, medium height and somewhat athletic. I think I'm a real figure woman."

"What is meant by "sexual body parts"? Can I see examples?"

"I'm a professional life drawing model and actress. The attached pic is pretty accurate for body type. Short waisted, big boobs & hips. BTW I'm 54, don't often cop to it."

"I am a 53 year-old real woman and my 'body parts' aren't so great - lots of nasty scars, etc."

"I'm 18, I'm a cheerleader and I go to school. I'm interested in being one of your models."

"I am interested in modeling for your study. I am 21 years-old, tall, slender & most definitely a real person..."

"Even as a nudist, finding nude woman can be tough. You may want to contact the local nudist resorts and ask to post on their web sites along with an explanation on what you're looking for and why."

"We are interested in posing, we are married and we love to be sexual, and show off. Attached a pic of a past event where we modeled [free-form body painting]."

Demographics

About The Photos

The breast photos herein are presented by age in decades, from smallest to largest in size. The women who posed for the pictures ranged in age from 18 to 70.

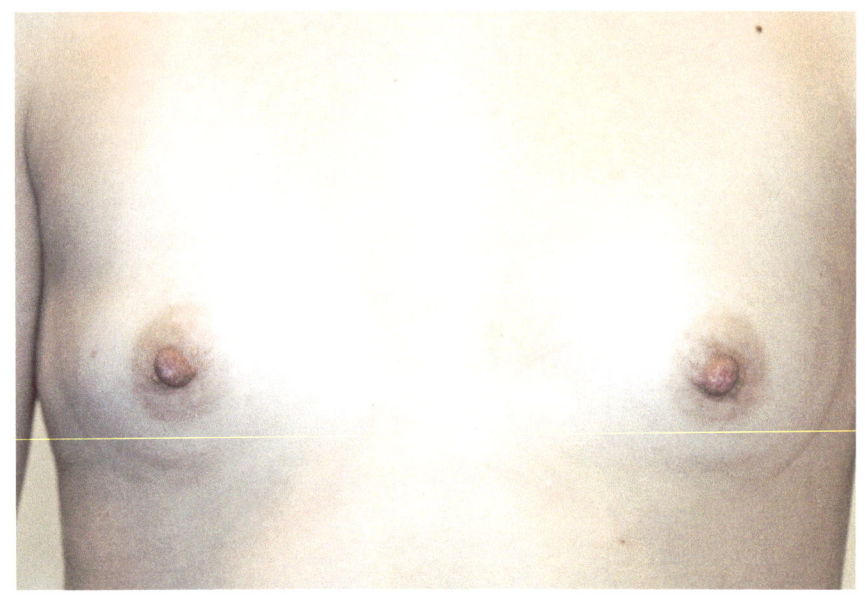

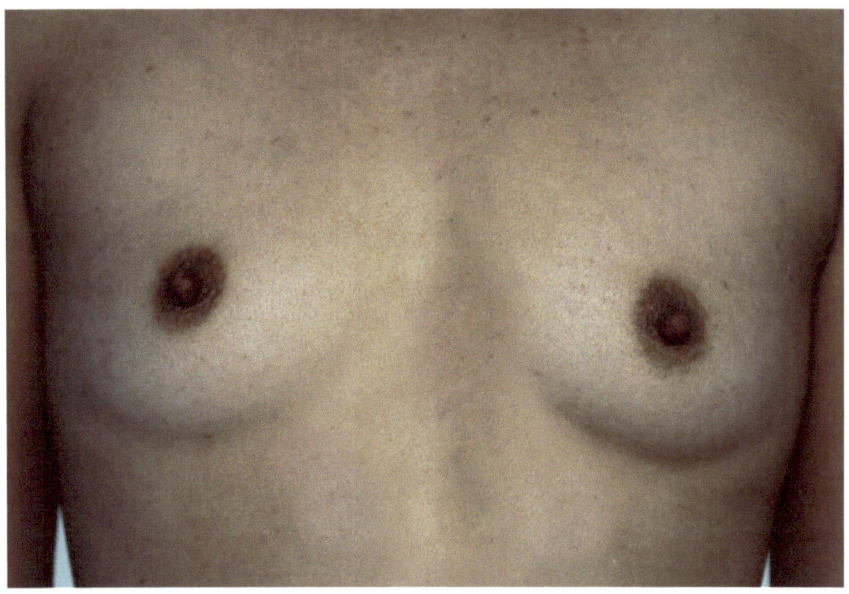

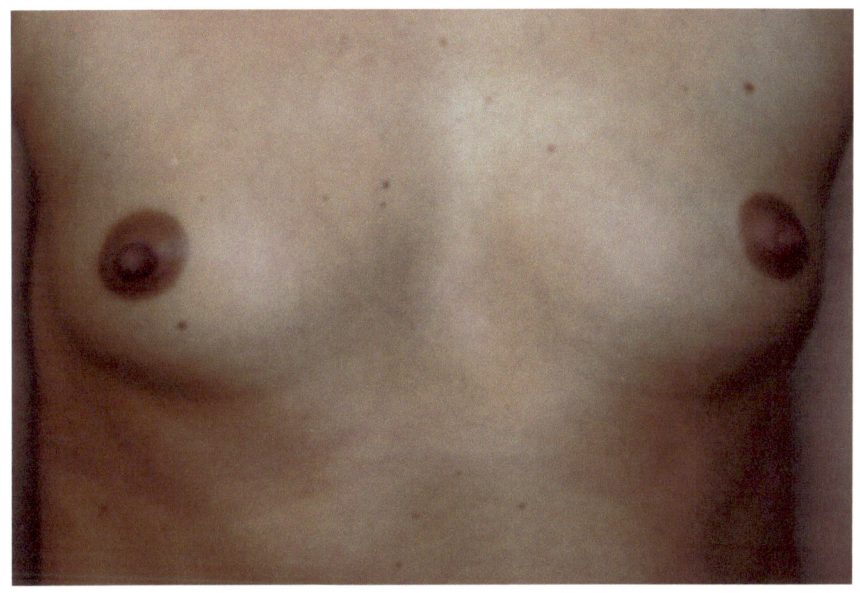

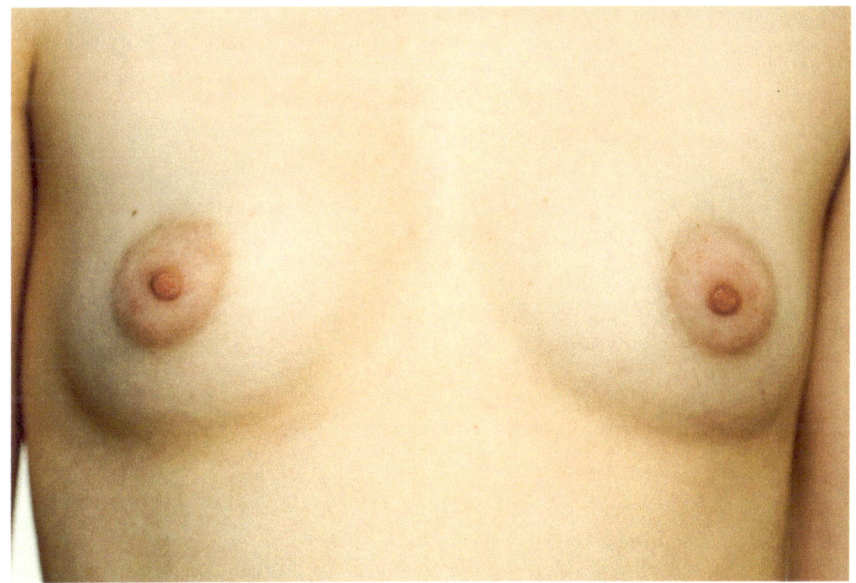

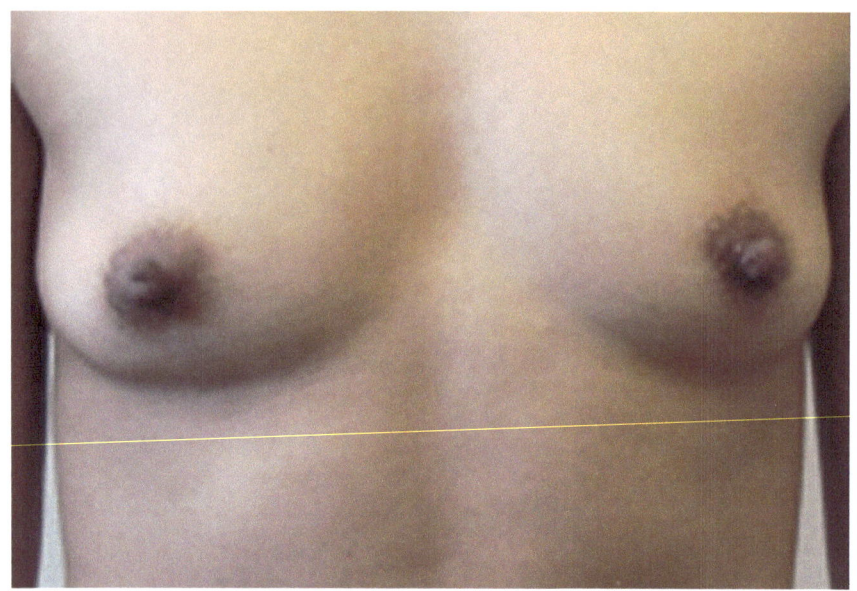

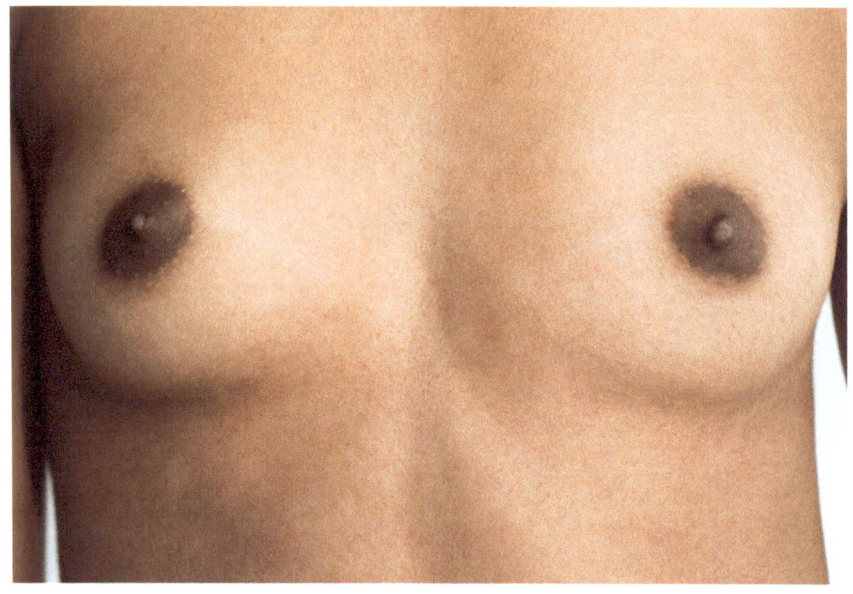

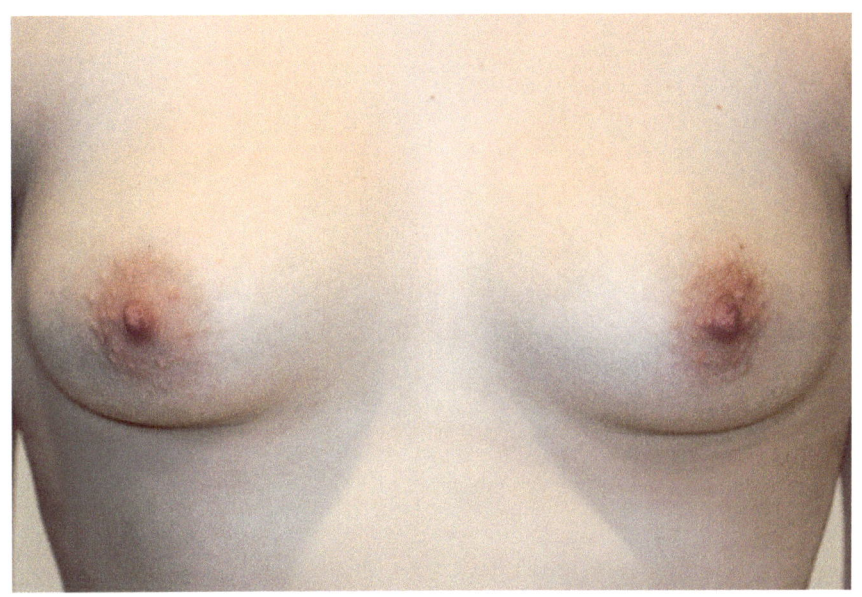

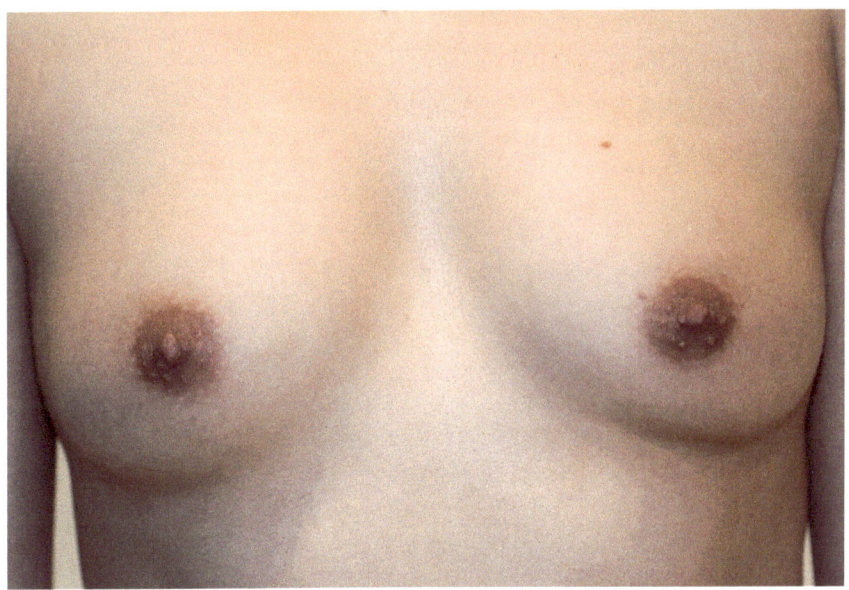

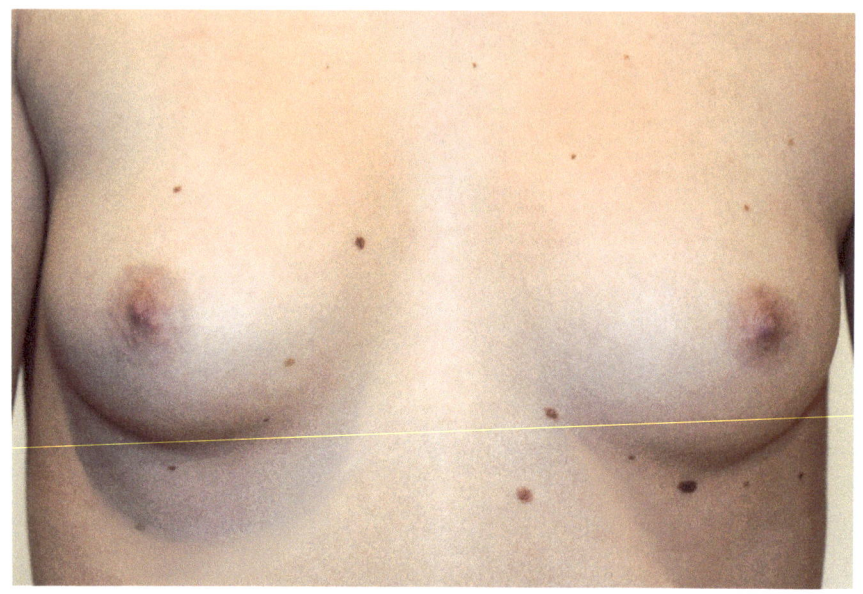

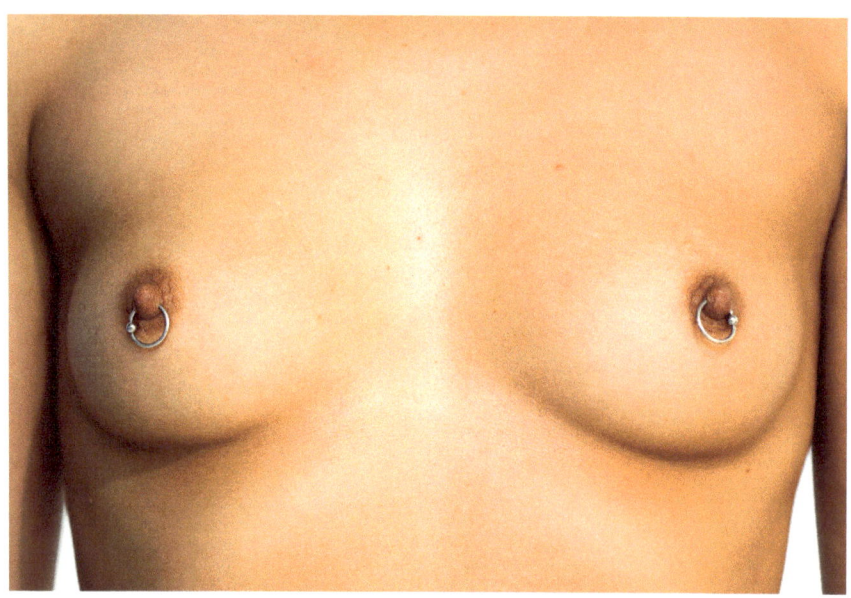

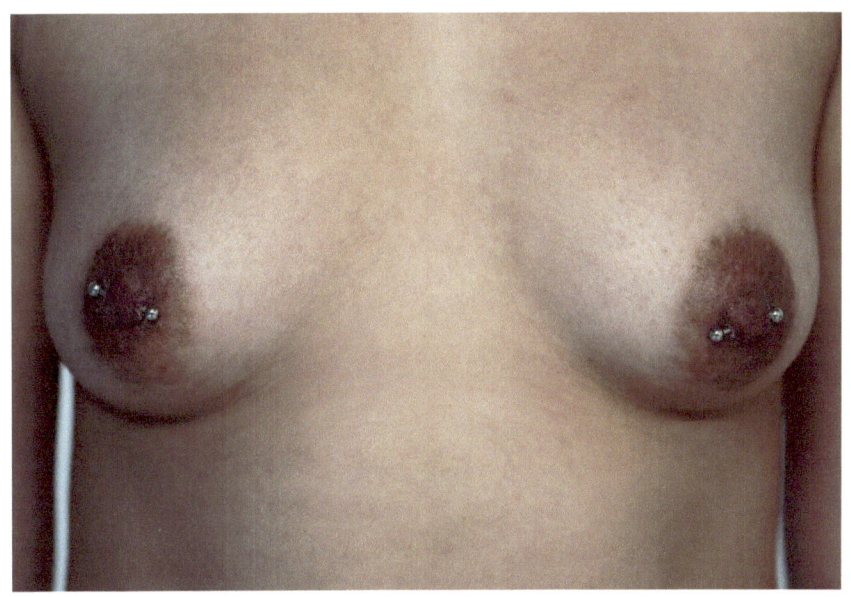

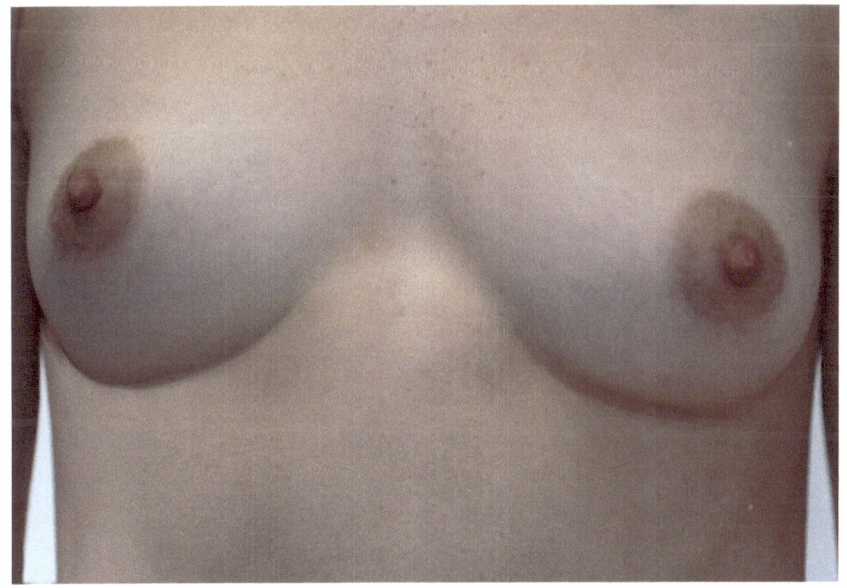

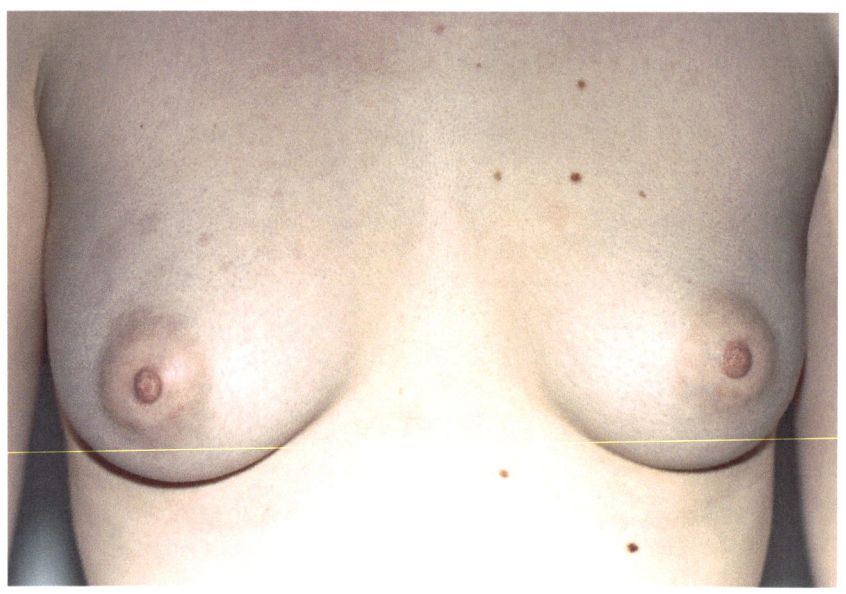

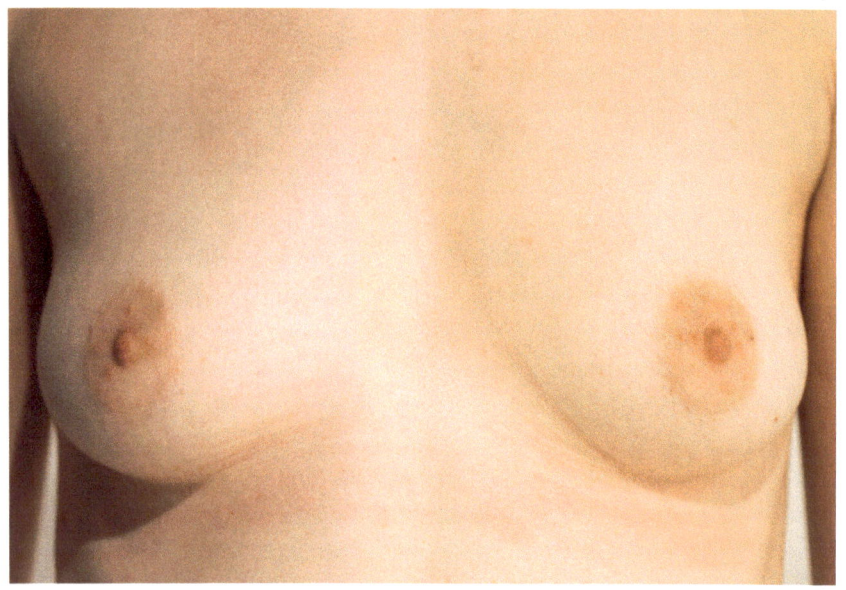

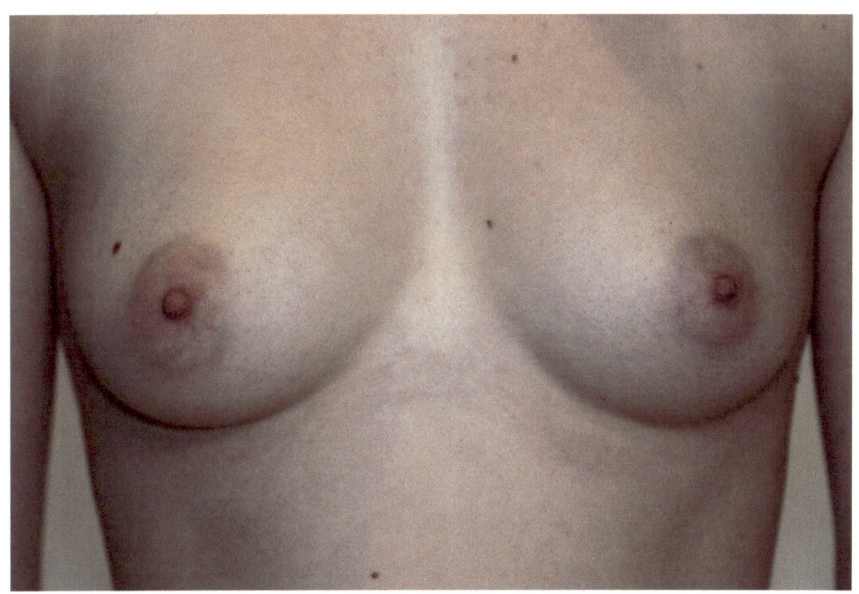

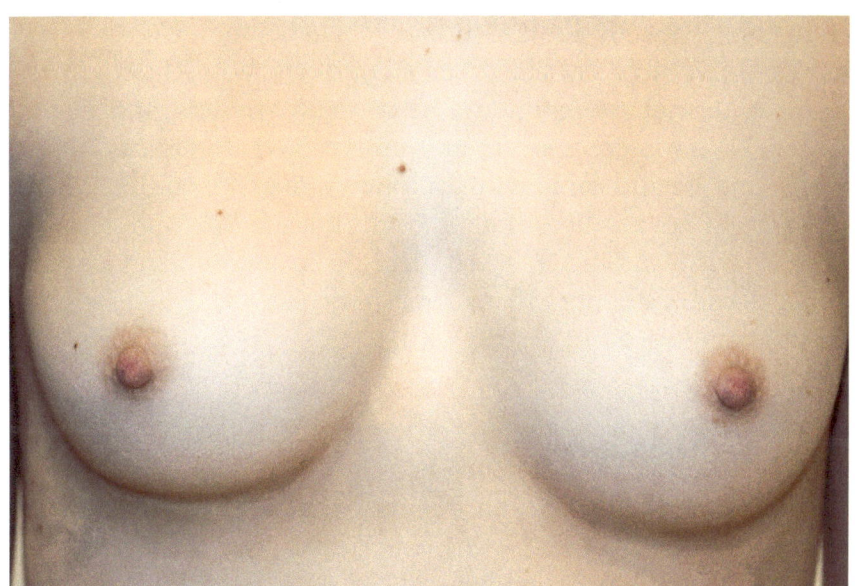

Who Are These Women?

Because I wanted to keep the relationships I developed in the artist enclave strictly professional, I decided to take selfies of my breasts for this publication. The process to photograph myself was hilarious but ultimately successful. After measuring the necessary height for the camera on its tripod stand, I affixed colored tape in the form of an "X" to both wall and floor, focused the camera, put the shutter on delayed release, ran to my spot, posed, calmed my breaths, and waited for the click. Needless to say, my photo required multiple takes.

The first woman who came into my studio was a French foreign exchange student working as a nanny while trying to break into modeling – young, lovely and at ease in her own skin. She observed that urban French and Continental European women had far fewer misgivings about their bodies than American women, and that they ate less and were generally slimmer than their American counterparts. Her youth and beauty came with an inherent arrogance that easily gives birth to a self-confident body image. She and I were close to the same cup size, yet I had three children and almost three decades on her. If my breasts now looked like hers, I would parade around topless with ease.

A well-dressed, well-spoken, older couple referred by studio management strolled in hand-in-hand. The gentleman spoke of their philosophy to find beauty in all life, while his wife expressed a desire that both men and women appreciate the wonders of the human body in all shapes, sizes and colors.

She said that her body definitely showed signs of her age... her husband put his arms around her and said she was even more beautiful at 60, than when he met her in her 20s. Men: take note.

Two college friends and soccer teammates came in together. Egging each other on, one claimed that her friend had perfect breasts. The young lady referred to was a self-professed tomboy who looked just that – her hair was short, her face free of makeup and her clothes androgynous. After the photo shoot, I had to agree that this woman had what many consider perfect breasts. The irony was she desperately wished she were an A cup instead. Her easy-going friend was lovely as well and completely comfortable in her own skin. She liked who she was and how she looked. What a refreshing attitude to see in Generation Y women.

An 18 year-old girl came in on the arm of her boyfriend. Her jeans were embroidered and there were flower appliqués on her purse. A barrette held back her bangs. She sent her beau out to the waiting area, turned to me and quietly said that she was very nervous but committed to participating in my photo shoot. We spoke about my desire for *The Private Square* to present the beauty and wonders of what normal women look like as well as the wondrous yet visible toll life, motherhood and the passage of time have on our bodies. She then told me that for as long as she could remember, she had always been a girl but her [physical] body was male. "It never has and never will represent my female soul". She asked if she could still be in my book. I said yes. *The Private Square* book series presents actual anatomy, so she and I agreed her photo would be in *Volume 1: Penises.* Even though she likely will never be able to afford hormone treatment or gender reassignment surgery, it was clear to me that she was a thoughtful and extraordinarily courageous young lady.

Breasts As Art

Through the ages, breasts have been associated with fertility and nourishment. As far back as ancient times, civilizations from every continent have examples of art that depict the feminine breast in this manner. The earliest example may be The Venus of Willendorf, a 30,000-22,000 years old statuette believed to have been made by the Ice Age Gravettian who dwelled in what is the present day northeastern border of Austria with the Czech Republic.

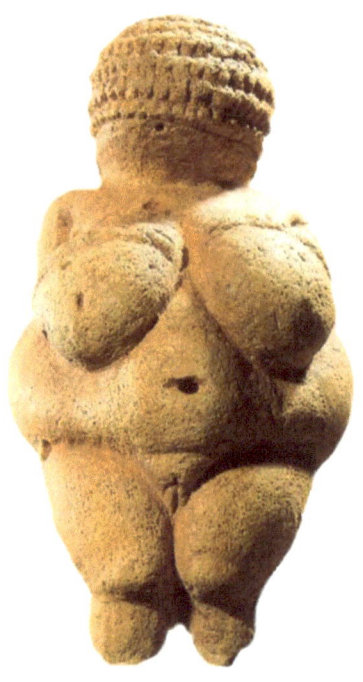 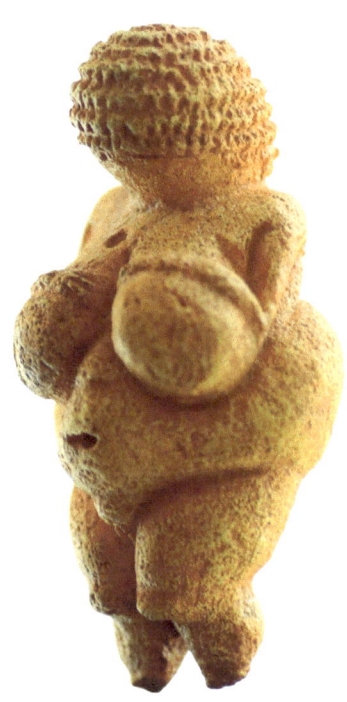

Note Artemis of Ephesus. Her legend dates back to 550 BCE when a temple dedicated to her honor was built in Ephesus (now modern day Turkey) by the Achaemenid dynasty of the Persian Empire. Greek Mythology said that Artemis was the daughter of Leto and Zeus, and the twin of Apollo. Among other things, she is the goddess of fertility. She is the helper of midwives as a goddess of birth. Many-breasted, she epitomizes female fertility and nourishing power.

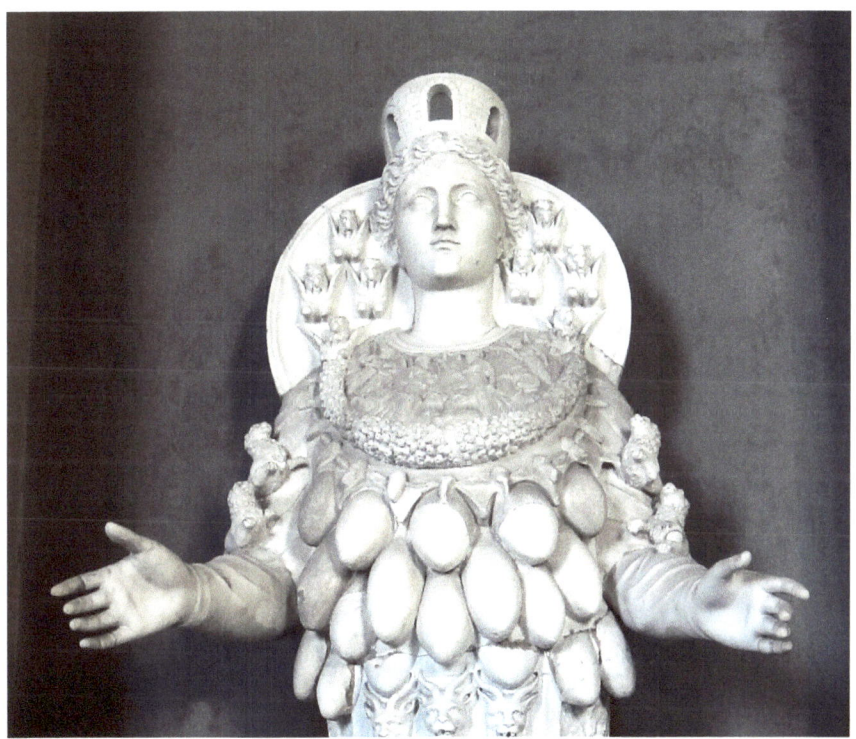

The Mahayana Buddhist Lotus Sutra was written sometime between 100 BCE and 100 CE and among other gods, featured Hariti, the Buddhist goddess for the protection of children. Note the infant nursing at her breast.

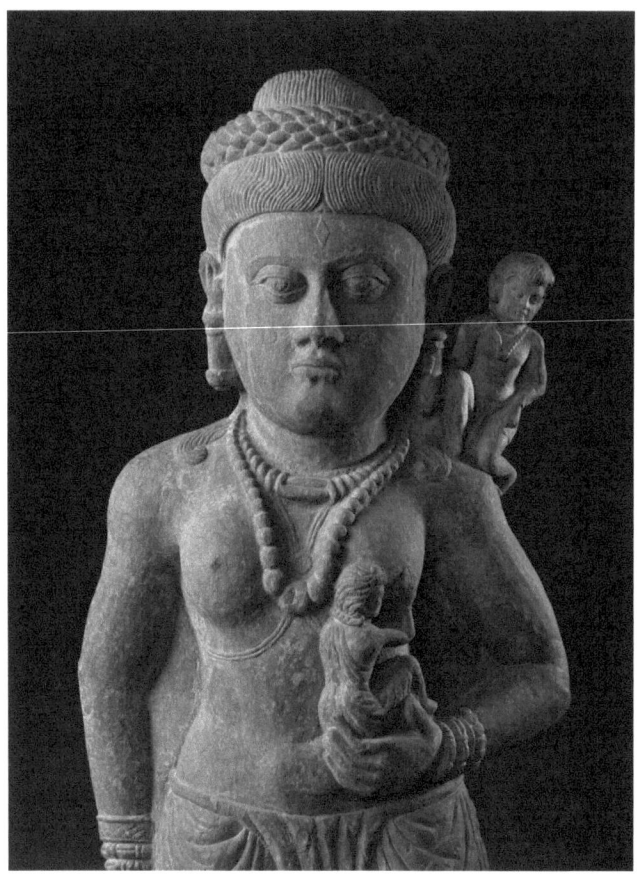

Sculpted around the turn of the Common Era, 100 BCE to 300 CE, another goddess was immortalized in marble – the Venus de Milo. Discovered in 1820, almost two millenium later, on the Greek Island of Melos her figure is considerably modernized from that of Artemis and Hariti.

During the Middle Ages, nudity was verboten. Women depicted in Christian paintings and sculptures were draped and clothed. The birth of the Renaissance and Age of Discovery, coupled with advances in science and medicine, led artists to focus on "humanism," and art through the 18th Century became more realistic. In much of the religious art of the time, female nudity alluded to motherhood.

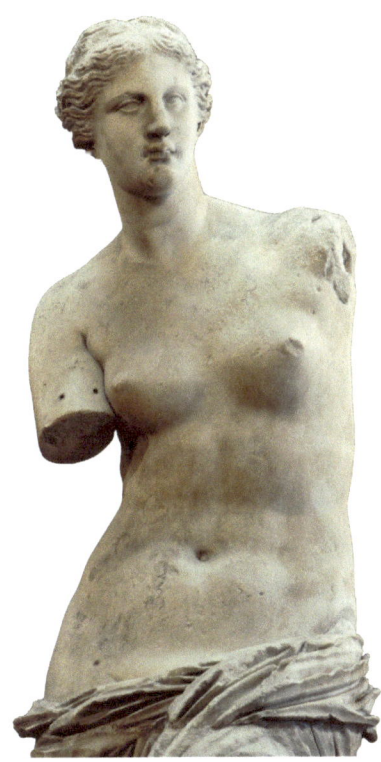

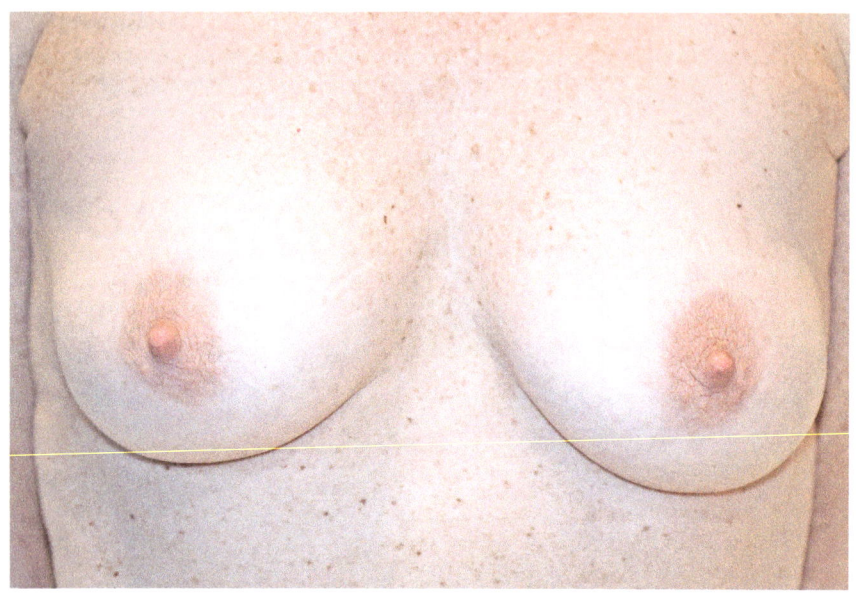

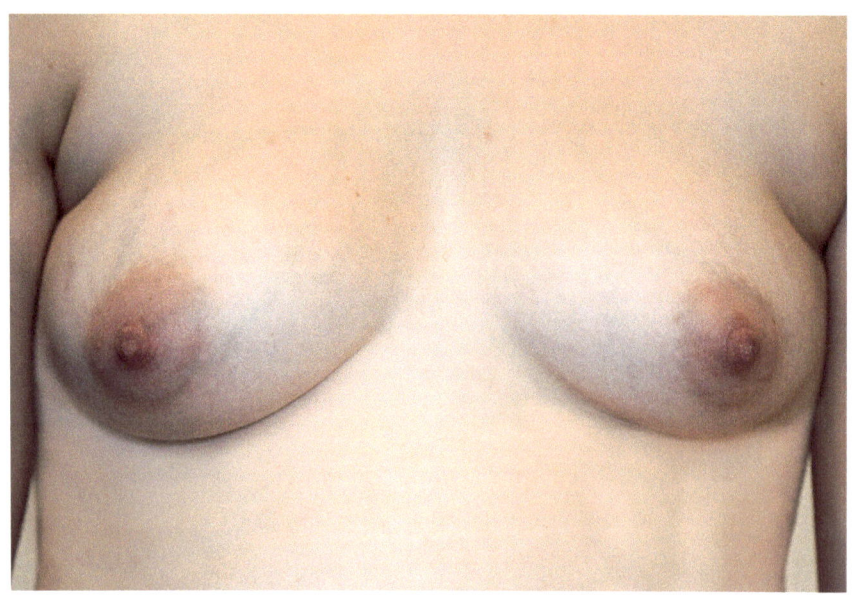

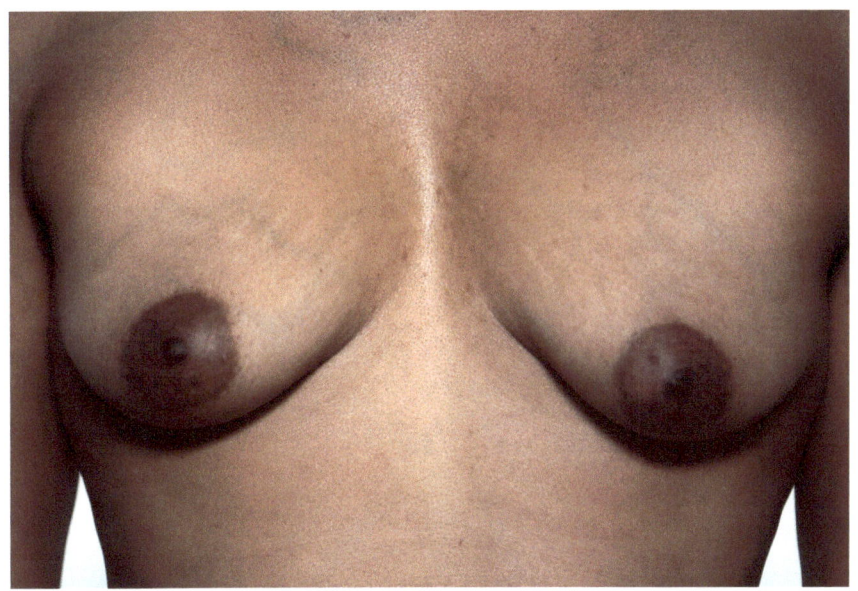

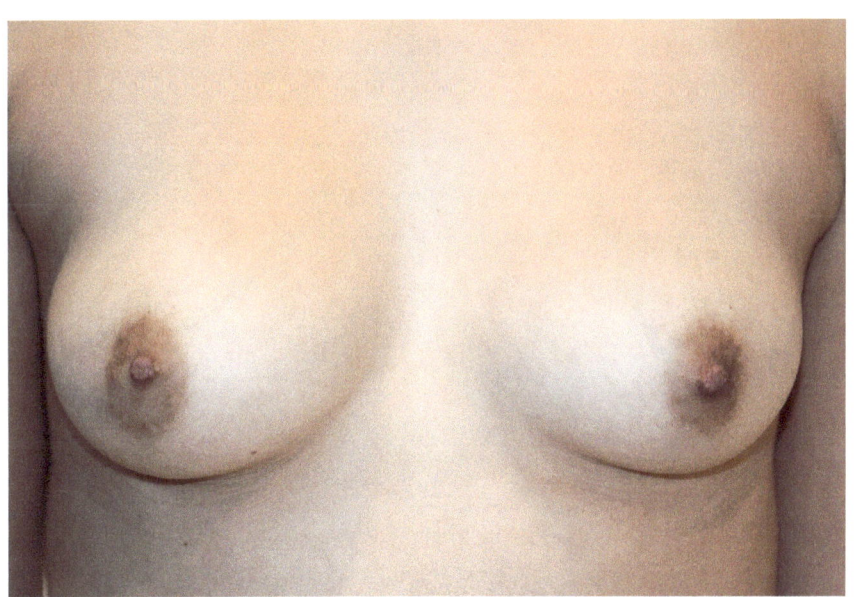

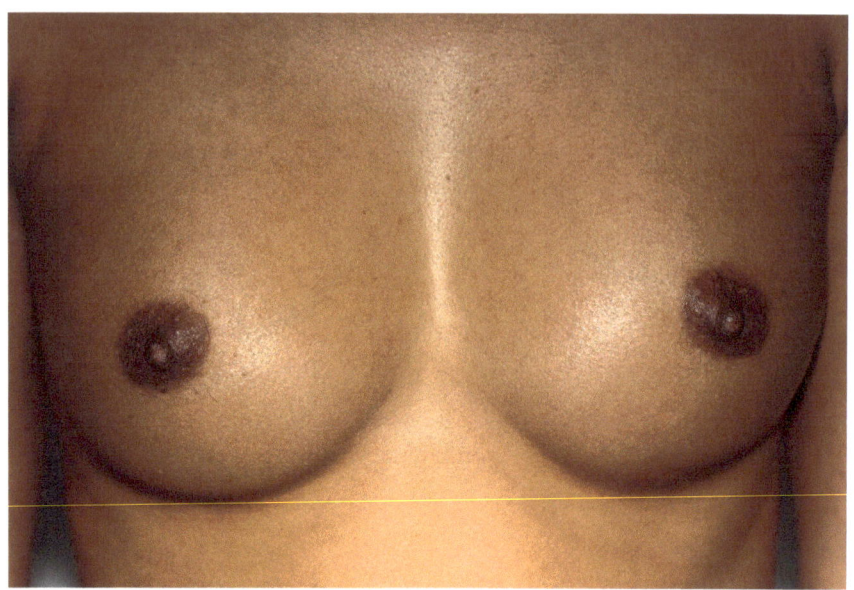

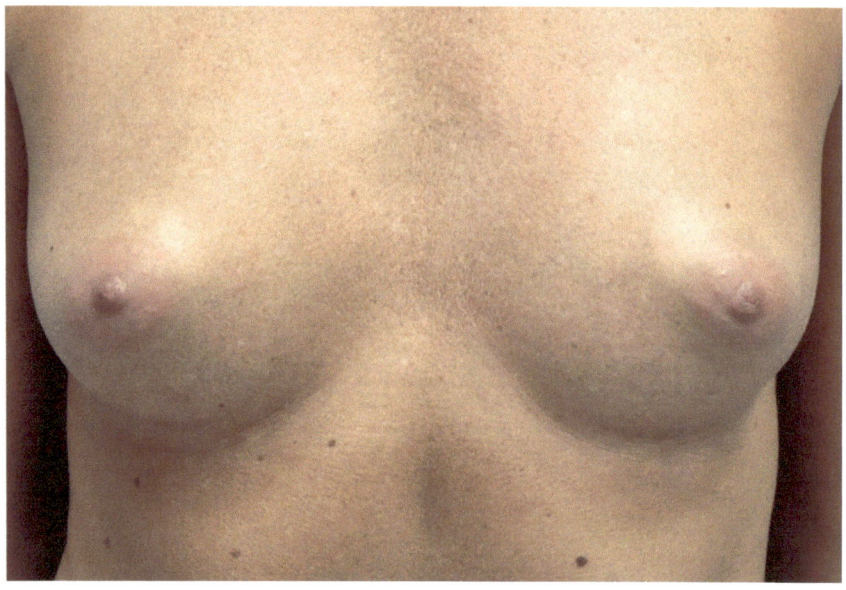

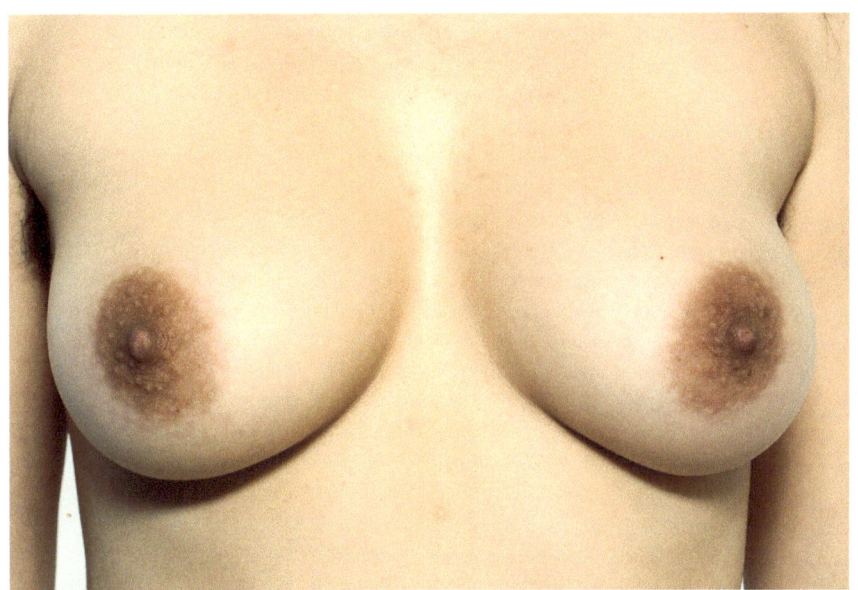

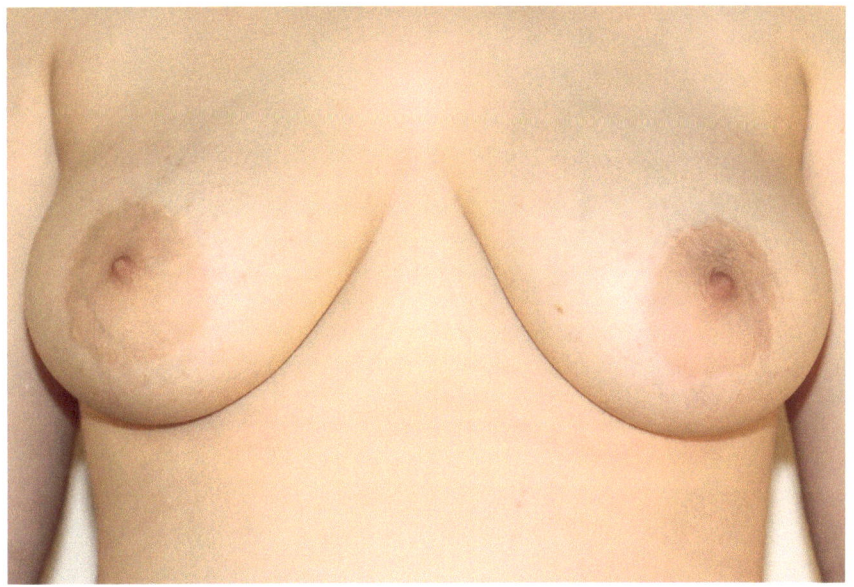

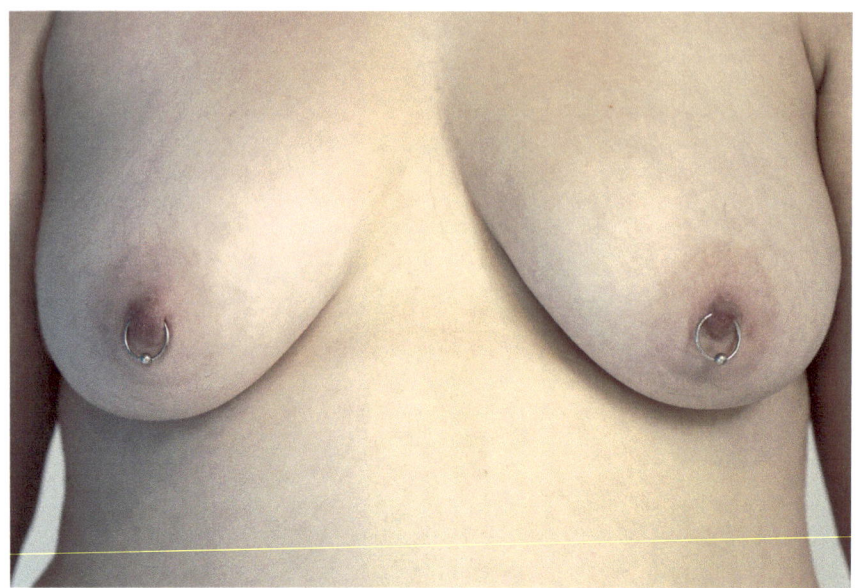

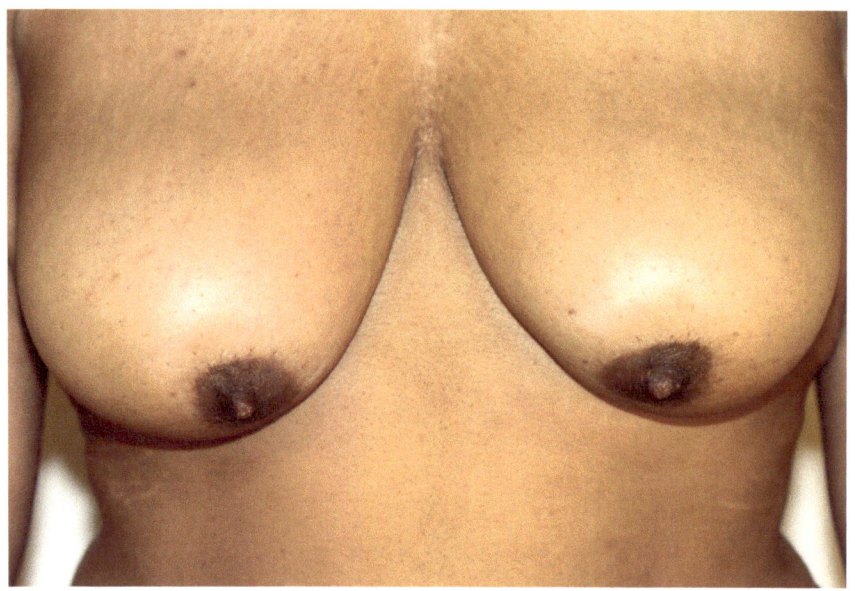

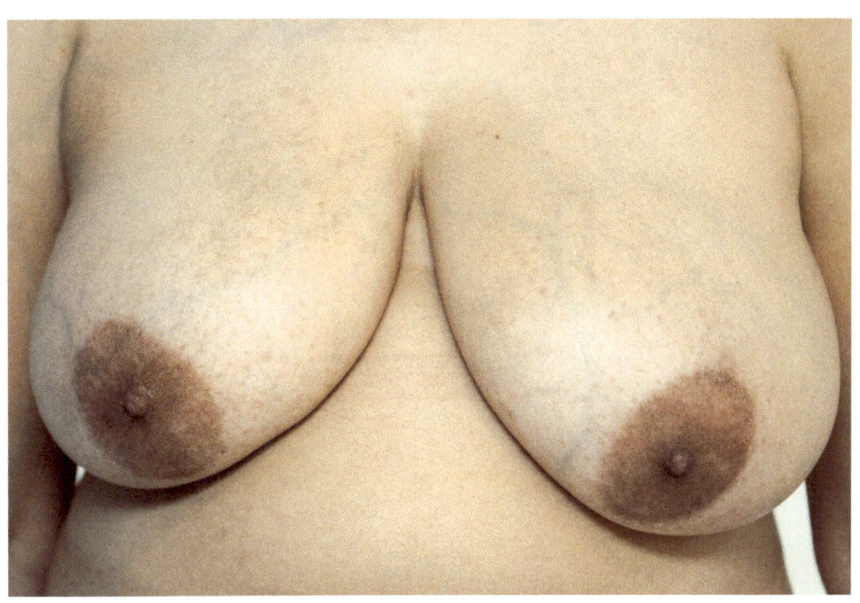

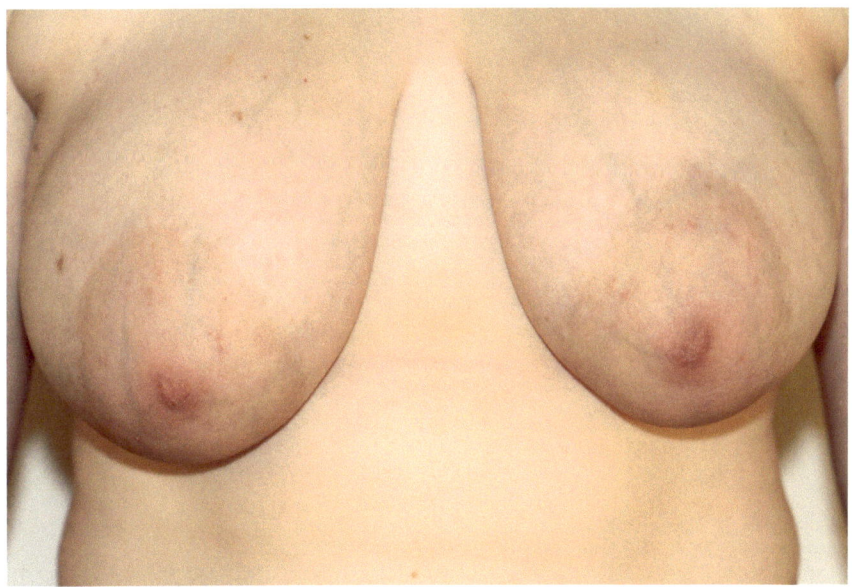

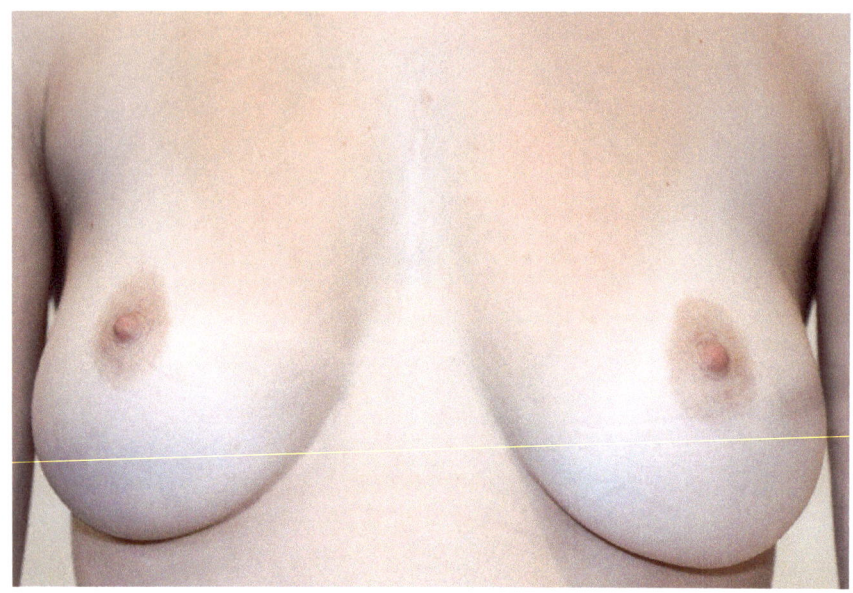

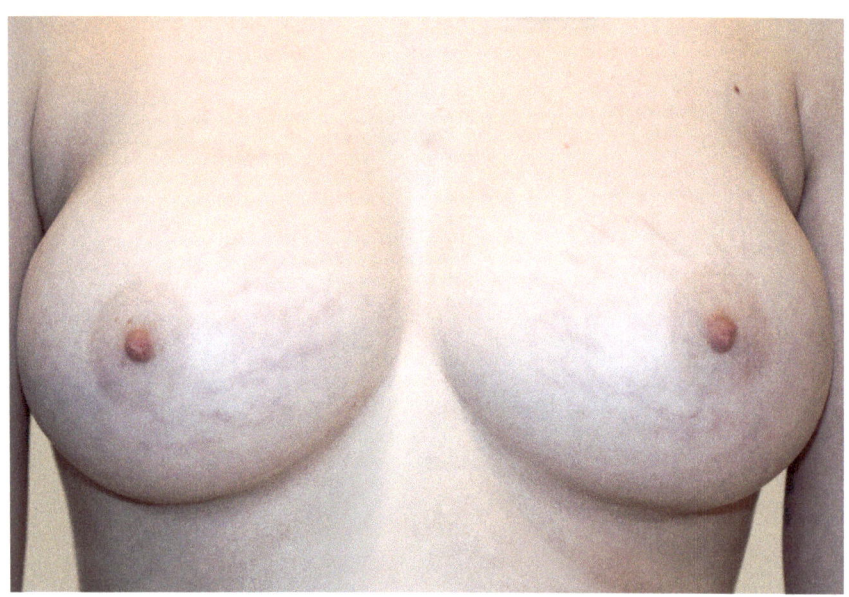

FROM CHESTS TO BREASTS

In the early stages of mammalian embryonic development, both females and males have thickenings of the skin in their chest known as the mammary ridge or milk lines. These milk lines extend from the inside of each upper arm down the torso and curve together in the genital area of the groin. As the fetus develops, these give rise to the mammary glands and nipples but otherwise are usually not visible at birth. For humans, the only external evidence of this developmental mammary tissue is the nipple – usually two.

A common occurrence, in approximately 10% of both male and female newborns, is supernumerary or accessory nipples. Oftentimes, they are passed off as a birthmark. These extra nipple(s) occur along the "milk line" from the breast to the pelvis. Usually, there will be one, maybe two ultra-small nipples – commonly mistaken for a mole. The most one of the long-time pediatricians I conferred with saw in his practice was a patient who had five accessory nipples.

Through childhood, breast tissue is no different in boys than in girls. At the onset of puberty things change. About the time a young girl is 9 to 11 years-old, her ovaries start secreting a hormone called estrogen. This causes fat to begin accumulating in the mammary ridge. A small lump will form under her nipple. This is called a breast bud. In rare cases, breast tissue can develop under supernumerary nipples – many who have this condition choose to have the excess surgically removed.

In some girls, breast development is cause for excitement, as they know they are entering the first phase of womanhood. Other girls may be horrified because the last thing they want is to give up their childhood or even be noticed. Almost every girl and mother has a story to tell about this phase of puberty. There was the girl who came to her mother complaining about a mosquito bite on her chest. Her nipple was swollen and red and it itched and felt funny. No bug bite, just a breast bud. Another girl cried for three weeks before pulling her mom into the bathroom, lifting her shirt and putting her mother's hand on her chest where a bump had formed. Three months later, when the second breast bud popped, she cried again - this time for only a week. One girl took to wearing her older sister's bra, stuffing the cup with tissue because her buds did not yet fill them out. Some girls, even parents, panic thinking the bump is some kind of abscess, tumor or cyst. Others ignore it and start wearing looser tee-shirts. Today, there are camisoles with built in shelf bras adding a second layer of fabric so that the girls' nipples are not showing through their shirts. And of course, they all start reading Judy Blume's *Are You There God? It's Me Margaret*, American Girl Publishers *The Care and Keeping of You: The Body Book for Girls* and more on the subject.

Some facts about early breast maturation: The breasts do not usually develop in a synchronized fashion. It is fairly common to get one breast bud and not see the other pop for weeks, even months. In the early stages of puberty as breasts develop they can be visibly different in size and shape. This difference typically subsides within a year, but as evidenced by the photos herein, most women do not have completely symmetrical breasts. Early breast tissue can be quite sensitive and some girls experience tenderness or other sensory symptoms.

The Five Stages Of Breast Development[1]

Stage One: pre-adolescent when only the tip of the nipples are raised on a girl's chest

Stage Two: appearance of breast buds, and slight enlargement of the nipples, areolae and breasts

Stage Three: breasts enlarge as more glandular breast tissue develops

State Four: areolae and nipples rise and protrude from breasts

Stage Five: breasts fill out, usually leaving only the nipples protruding

Breasts respond to the levels of estrogen in the body. During the first half of a woman's menstrual cycle, the ovaries release estrogen to prepare a woman for pregnancy. The estrogen causes the milk ducts to enlarge and girls/women might feel their breasts become tender or lumpy during this phase of their cycle. Prior to ovulation, a hormone called progesterone is released that causes the uterine lining to thicken.

If conception occurs, the sustained hormonal stimulation will cause the areola to darken and the entire breast to swell as the milk ducts increase in size. Breast tenderness and swelling is often the first sign of pregnancy. Breasts continue to respond to pregnancy. The increase in size and circulation cause increased vascularization and blood vessels become more visible. By the end of the second trimester the breasts are capable of producing milk. Further in her life cycle, as a woman enters menopause (the complete cessation of her menstrual cycle), estrogen production is significantly reduced. Over time, this results in a reduction in the glandular breast tissue and a degradation of the connective tissue therein.

Breasts lose shape, shrink and sag – how much it affects the aesthetic of the breasts depends in part on personal genetics and how much adipose (fat) tissue is present. It happens to every woman.

On that note, it is time to address men's breasts. Yes, men have breasts but they do not develop in the same manner women's do. For virtually all boys and men, they do not develop in the same manner as women's breasts do. During their first two weeks of life, baby girls and baby boys can have swelling of the nipple. A few babies even have a nipple discharge sometimes called "witch's milk." The condition is medically known as galactorrhea and is the result of the mother's hormones still circulating in the infant's blood stream. It usually resolves within two weeks.

As with girls, puberty is when boys' bodies begin to change. Early in puberty, most boys will have some breast tenderness. During puberty, more than half of boys develop some swelling of breast tissue – this pudginess is different than the excess fat heavier boys have on their chest. Most of the time, the swelling is no more than one centimeter. However, it is not uncommon for boys to think they have a tumor or something else seriously wrong with them.

Many pediatricians and family physicians purposely point out this developmental milestone to their male patients in order to lessen the anxiety that accompanies this stage of physical development. The condition is called Gynecomastia[2] and it is caused by inconsistent and changing levels of androgens, the predominant male hormones which lead to the development of characteristics like deeper voices, hair growth and increased muscle size. The most well known androgens being the hormones testosterone and far less known to men, estrogen.

Note: Men and women have both androgen and estrogen produced by a variety of glands in the body (hypothalamus, pituitary, adrenal) in addition to hormones produced in the testes and ovaries. Gynecomastia normally resolves over a period of months to two years. In rare cases, the breast tissue will develop further than a little swelling into what looks like female breast. In those instances, most boys elect to have the tissue surgically removed.[3] In 2013, of the total reported breast surgeries performed worldwide, almost 8% were for gynecomastia.[4]

Since men have breasts per se, they can also get breast cancer. One percent of the incidences of breast cancer in the United States per year are in men. In contrast, breast cancer is the most common cancer worldwide in women contributing more than 25% of the total number of new cancer cases diagnosed annually. Women who have had more than one close relative diagnosed with breast cancer may have inherited a mutated gene identified as BRCA1 or BRCA2. Compared to women in the general population, who have a 7% risk of developing breast cancer by age 70, the average risk of developing breast cancer for women with the BRCA1 gene is 55%-65%, and for BRCA2 carriers 45%-47%. Factors associated with a decreased risk of breast cancer include breastfeeding for at least one year, regular moderate or vigorous physical activity, and maintaining a healthy body weight.[5]

For more than 50 years, the medical community has endorsed breast self-exams (BSE).[6] Cancer organizations, medical institutes and health care providers first propagated a circular palpitation of each breast from a standing or prone position, and most recently a vertical grid-search multi-pressure methodology while lying flat on one's back to feel for lumps, bumps or other changes in one's own breast tissue. Your healthcare provider can provide instructions for these methods, or they are easily found online. In 2009, The United States Preventative Services Task Force, and separately, the Canadian Task Force on Preventative Health, cited evidence that regular BSE do not reduce breast cancer deaths but do lead to an increase in anxiety and unnecessary procedures.

Subsequently, in 2015 many health authorities are advocating for "breast self-awareness" which encourages women (and men) to be mindful of what their breasts normally look and feel like so that they can inform their physician if there are any physical changes. The general consensus of health care organizations for women without a family history of breast cancer is the following:

Women in their 20s and 30s should get clinical breast exams every three years.

Women in their 40s who have a family history of cancer should begin getting annual mammography screening exams. Women with no family history should discuss clinical breast cancer screening with their physician to consider getting a baseline mammogram some time in their 40s and screening mammograms every 2-3 years through age 49.

Women 50 years and older should have a mammogram every two years.

Some women, approximately 2% of the population, "because of their family history, genetic tendency or certain other factors should be screened with MRI in addition to mammograms."[6]

For both women and men, any reddening, darkening or swelling, puckering, scaliness, sores, new and persistent pain or lump on or around the breast area, including the nipple and armpits OR any physical change in the nipple including discharge, is cause for concern and should be seen by a medical doctor as soon as possible. Men – that means call your doctor immediately and ask for an urgent appointment. If it is past office hours call anyway and leave a message.

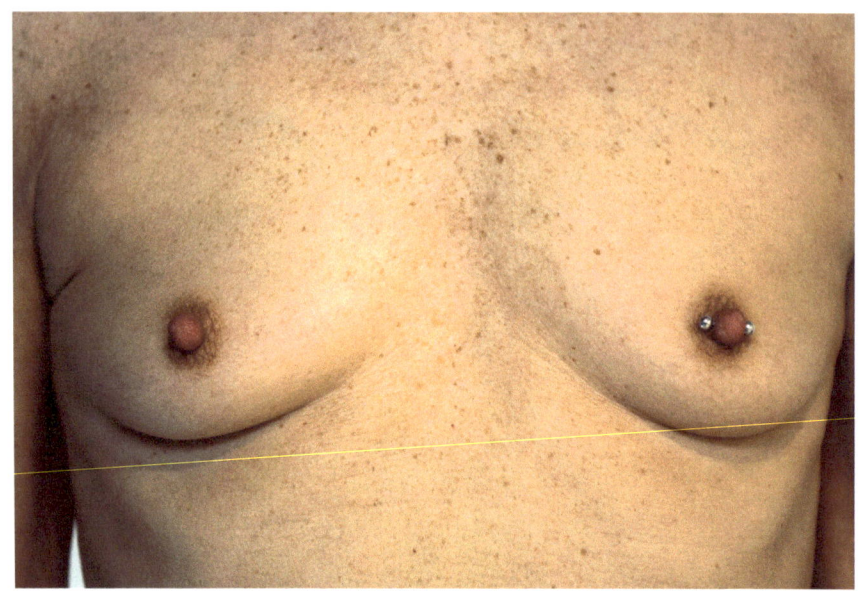

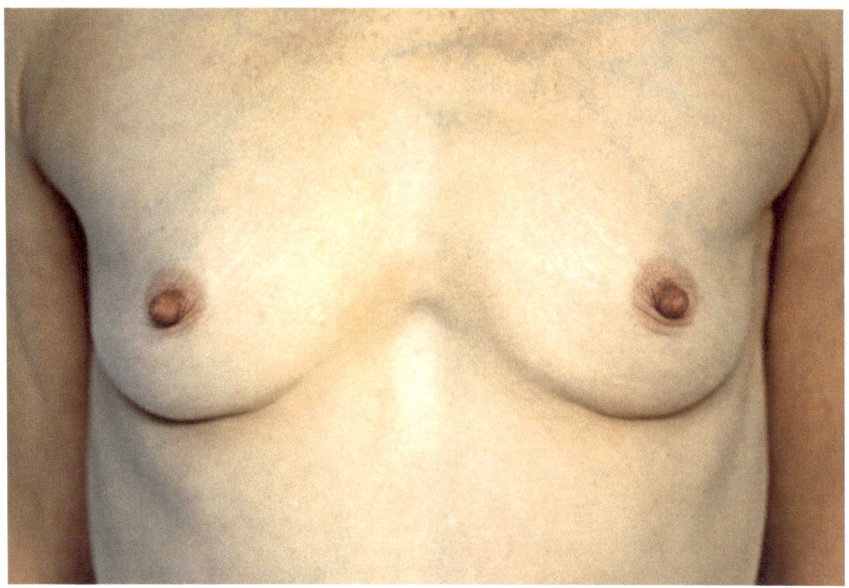

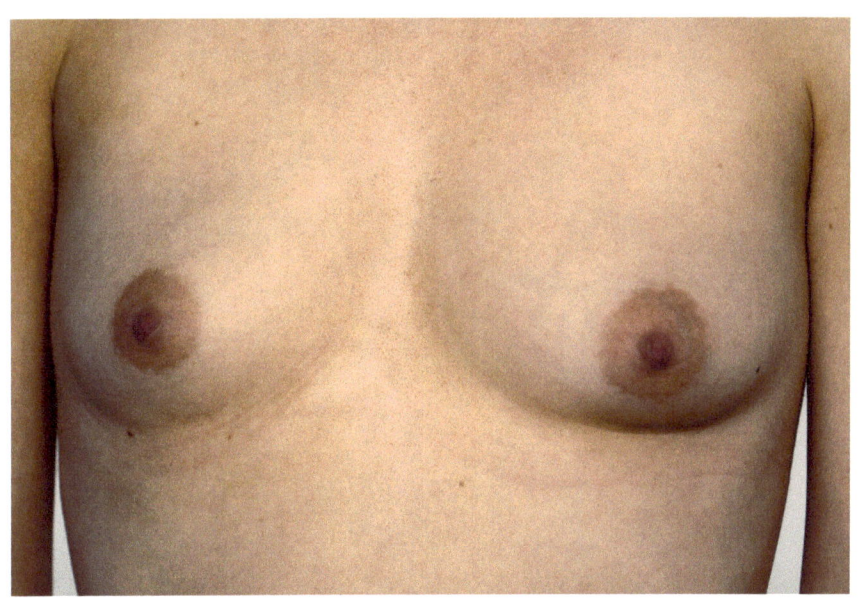

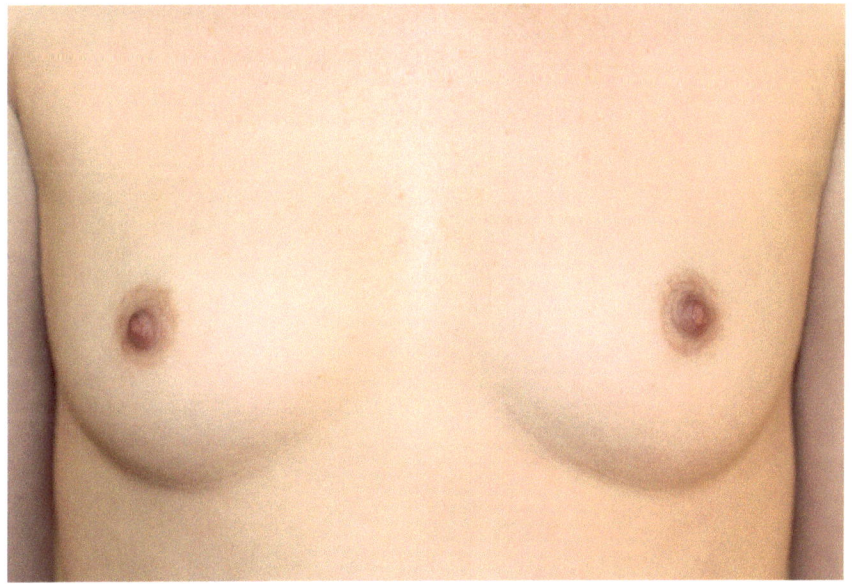

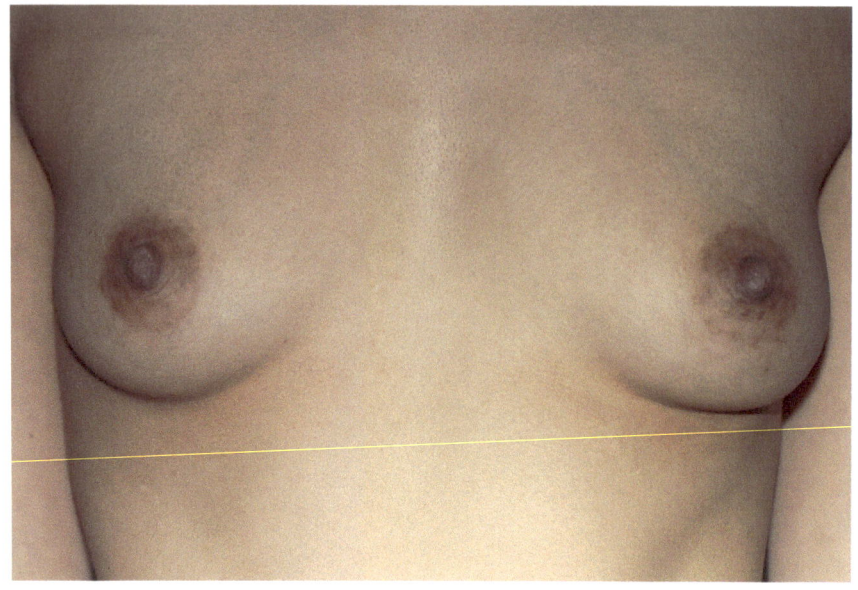

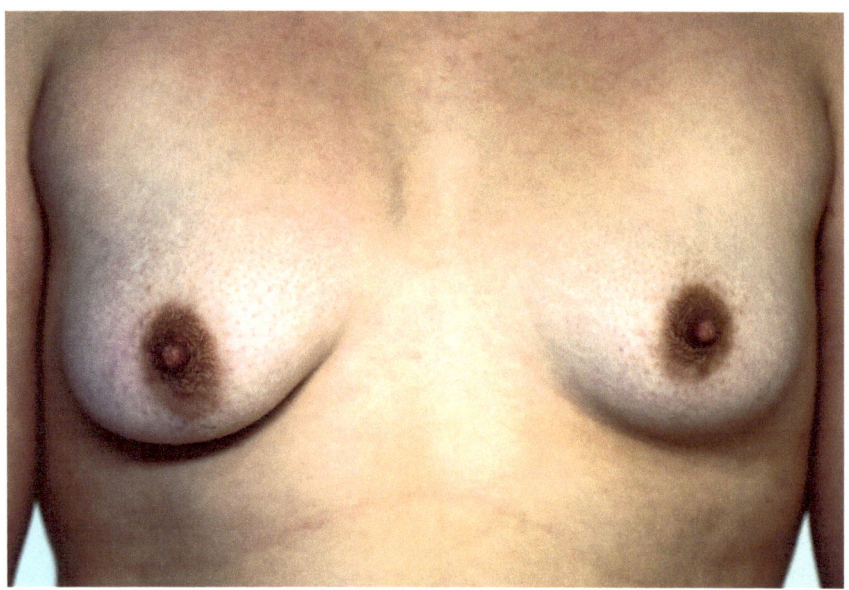

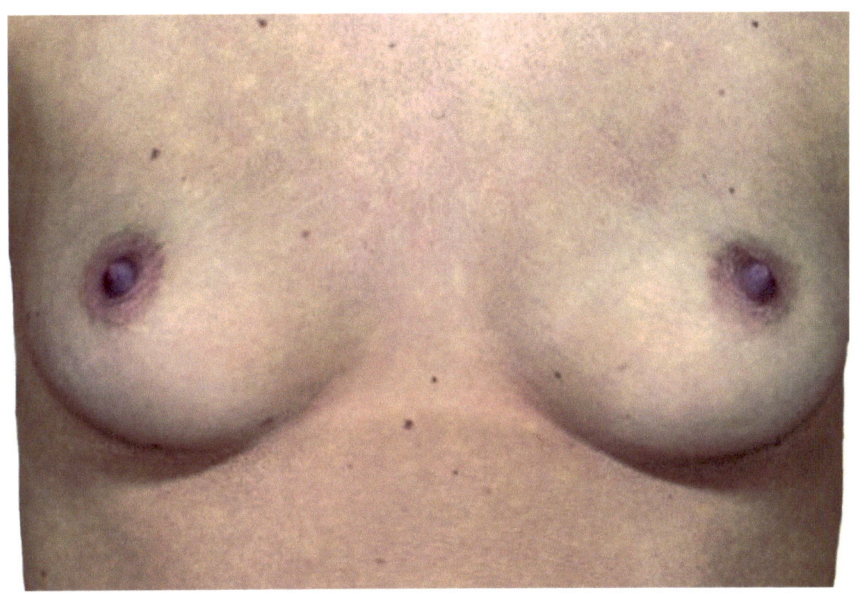

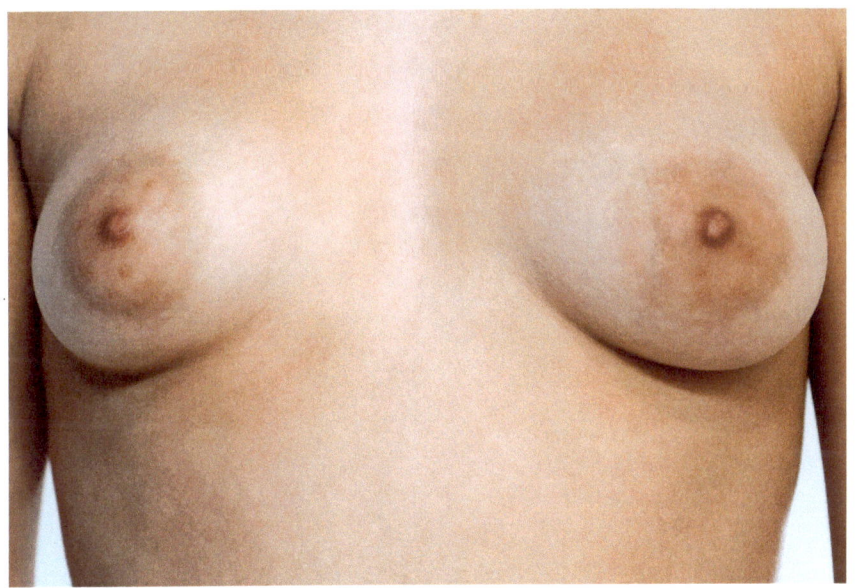

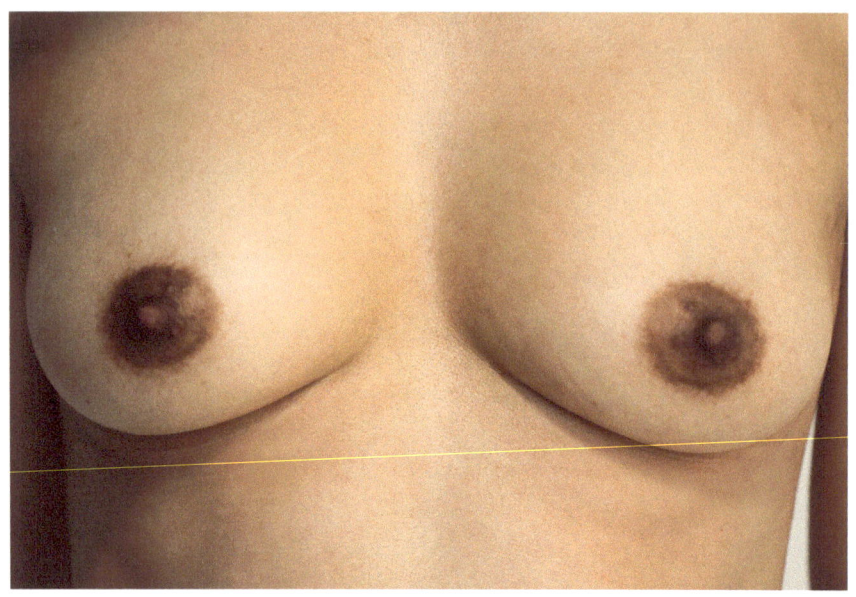

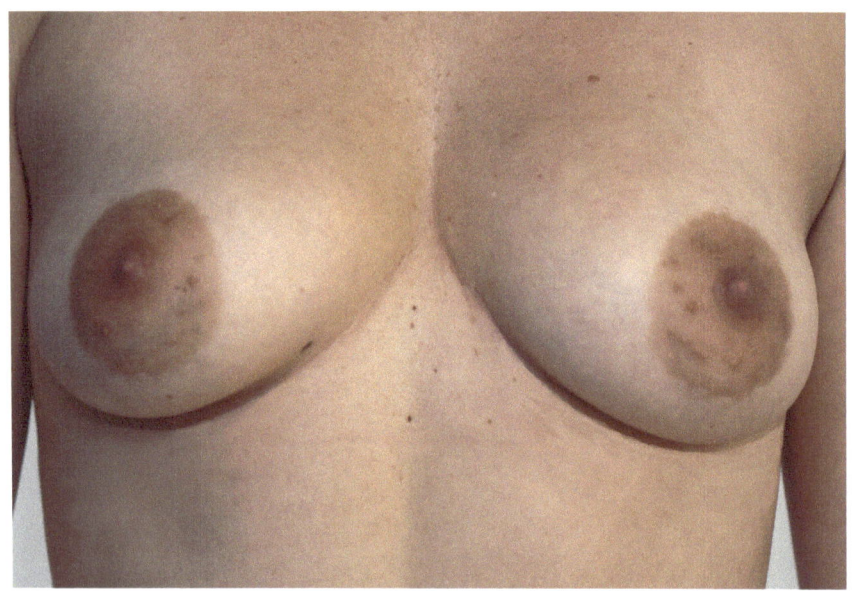

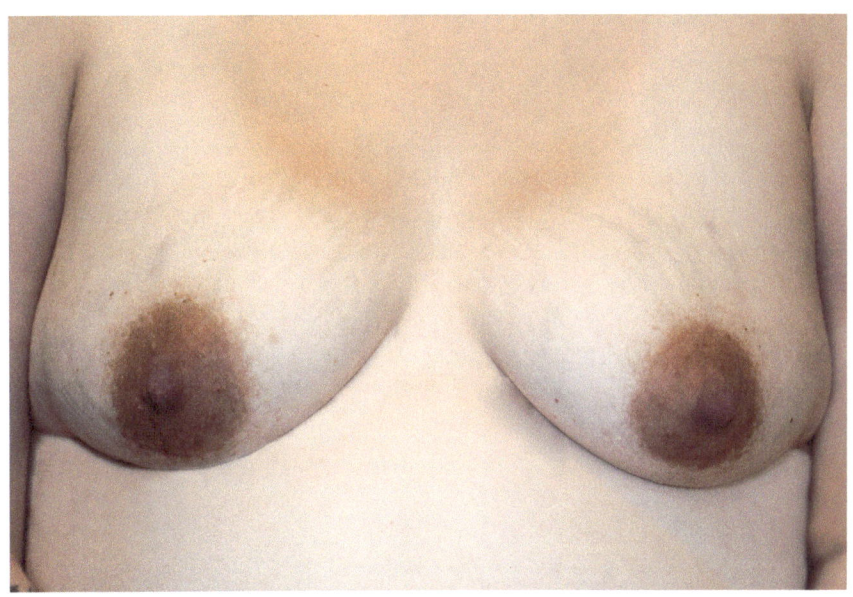

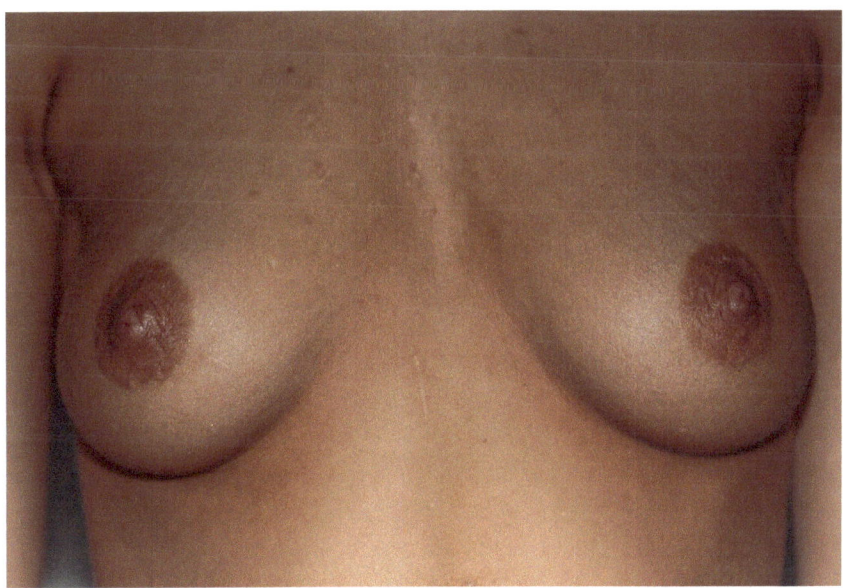

Who Are These Women? continued

Contrary to my experience photographing men during T*he Private Square Volume 1: Penises,* many women came to my studio in pairs. There is clearly bravery and safety in sisterhood. One such pair had been friends for more than thirty years – since high school. The first, a 49 year-old, was enthused enough to fling off her shirt, pose and have us check out her tits. Admittedly childless, she was quite proud and pleased how her breasts had stood the test of time. She was sincerely complimentary of her friend, a mother of two preteens, who willingly posed for the camera without any such preening.

A young woman I photographed was five months pregnant. Two other women were post-partum – one was still nursing her infant and the other had already weaned her six month-old baby. A visual reminder that women's bodies are designed for motherhood; our breasts are first and foremost a means to feed our young and that sexuality associated with breasts is more social than biological.

There was a six-foot tall coed who told me her breasts budded when she was twelve years-old and thereafter never grew. She had no choice but to wear padded, push-up bras because that was the only way to fill out clothes. Though she knew she was a candidate for a breast augmentation, at 22 years-old she had the poise and self-confidence to say: "This is me. Take it or leave it." If she ever decided to get a boob job, she said, it would be because she wanted it not because any guy told her she should get one.

Just three of my "models" had breast implants. It was obvious for one of the women when she was dressed that she had had implants due to the round, half dome shape her breasts took on when compressed by a bra. When her breasts were uncovered, however, they did not look at all like classic silicone enlargements. Post-op, she had an infection in one breast that, when healed, resulted in a slight but visible variance in the size and shape of that breast. She opted not to have a second surgery and healed nicely. Naked, her breasts look completely real. The second woman, clothed, did not look like she had implants. When she undressed however, the shape of her breasts, their position on her chest and the faint scars of a breast lift all indicated she had an augmentation. And the third woman opted for a smaller size implant and looked quite natural both in and out of clothes.

A college freshman who spoke with the maturity of a young woman well beyond her years posed for me. As with almost all adolescents, her breasts had an impact on her self-image and, with respect to potential relationships with boys, her self-worth. She believed that her sisters and seemingly all their friends had really nice breasts but not her. For an unknown reason, only one of her breasts fully developed leaving her at 16 years-old with one breast a size A and the other a "saggy" D cup. Fortunately for her, she came from a family with the means to pay for breast enlargement surgery using a technique called autologous fat transfer so that she did not have to have recurring surgery to replace implants every decade or so. Eighteen months later, her breasts are healed, virtually to the same size, but vary a bit in shape. Though slight differences in the size and shape of a woman's breasts is common and normal, she still struggled with self-image issues.

ARE THEY REAL?

Augmentation Mammoplasty is known commonly as breast implants and colloquially as a boob job. The objective of the surgery is to increase the fullness and projection of the breasts. Oftentimes, due to the spherical shape of many implants and the fact that surgically enhanced breasts appear higher on the chest than they normally would be for even an adolescent female, it is easy to tell whose are "fake" and whose are real. Medical device companies have begun to provide tear-drop shaped implants which are definitely more natural looking than their round counterparts.

The history of breast augmentation dates back to the mid-twentieth century.[7] In the 1940s, Japanese prostitutes enlarged their breasts by having them injected with paraffin, sponges or non-medical grade silicon because they believed American GIs found larger breasts more desirable. Silicone breast implants were developed by plastic surgeons Frank Gerow, MD and Thomas Cronin, MD, and in 1962, Timmie Jean Lindsey became the first woman to receive them. (There were also saline-filled implants, originated in 1964 by Laboratories Arion in France, but due to issues with deflation, these implants were a less popular choice amongst surgeons and women.) In 1976, the United States Congress passed the Medical Devices Amendment to the Federal Food, Drug and Cosmetic Act. This legislation gave the FDA the authority to review and approve the safety and effectiveness data of new medical devices. At this point, silicone breast implants had been on the market for almost 15 years, so they were "grandfathered" as approved under the new law.

Manufacturers of the implants were then required to provide product, side effect and areas of concern data... [only] when called to do so by the FDA.

Ralph Nadar's Citizen Health Research Group in Washington, DC sent out a warning bulletin that breast implants caused cancer in 1982. This resulted in the FDA proposing to recategorize silicone breast implants as a Class III medical device that required manufacturers to prove their safety in order to continue sales of these products. A 1984 lawsuit, Stern vs. Dow Corning, concluded that there was a connection between silicone-induced problems and subsequent autoimmune disease. Finally, in 1988, the FDA passed the legislation making silicone implants a Class III medical device and gave manufacturers three years to submit their FDA mandated Premarket Approval Application that required valid scientific data that proved their implants were safe. The FDA then had six months to review and confirm the manufacturers' findings in order to approve public sale thereof.[7]

The national media shined the spotlight on potential health problems related to the ever-growing popularity of silicone breast implants by airing a story on Face to Face with Connie Chung in December of 1990. By 1992, the FDA banned virtually all silicone filled breast implants. There was more than a decade of lawsuits, trials, and bankruptcy-causing settlements for some silicone implant makers as well as increasingly detailed government, professional, academic and international research into whether there was a connection between the implants and auto-immune or other illnesses. At the behest of the U.S. Congress, the Institute of Medicine, under the auspices of the esteemed National Academy of Sciences, formed an investigative committee to consider the safety of silicone breast implants.

In June 1999 the committee released a 400-page report prepared by a committee of 13 independent scientists. These experts examined past research and conducted public hearings. They concluded that surgeries associated with silicone breast implants may be responsible for localized problems such as hardening or scarring of breast tissue, but the implants themselves do not cause any major diseases such as cancer, lupus or rheumatoid arthritis.[8] The FDA allowed silicone gel-filled breast implants back on the market in November 2006 with the requirement that manufacturers conduct follow-up studies on their long-term safety. They approved their use for breast augmentation in women 22 or older, and for reconstructive surgery for women of any age. Furthermore, they note that these implants are not lifetime devices. According to the United Kingdom's National Health Service, and some implant manufacturers, after having breast implant surgery, about one in three women will require further surgery within 10 years of their initial operation.[9,10] And, the three major U.S. manufacturers only warranty their implants for 10 years.[10,11,12]

Recent statistics gathered by the International Society of Plastic Surgery show that in 2013 almost 3.5 million breast procedures were recorded, accounting for 30% of total cosmetic surgeries worldwide. With respect to breast enlargement or improvement surgery as a percent of the total, about 21% of Iranian and Mexican women had these procedures, while more than 34% of U.S. and Venezuelan women, followed closely by 32% of Brazilian women who elected for cosmetic surgery, had a breast augmentation, breast lift or breast reduction surgery in that year.[5] Mannequin makers in Venezuela actually redesigned their fiberglass females to mirror the extravagant bosom so many women were paying to get.[13] Life imitating art, or, art imitating life?

For the curious, three of the women photographed for this publication have implants – they are pictured on the bottom of Page 24, the top of Page 67, and the bottom of Page 82. The first two had augmentation mammoplasty (implants), and the third had both a mastopexy (breast lift) and augmentation.

The women whose bodies are pictured in the top photo on Page 24 and the bottom photo on Page 28 have had no surgery – their breasts are natural.

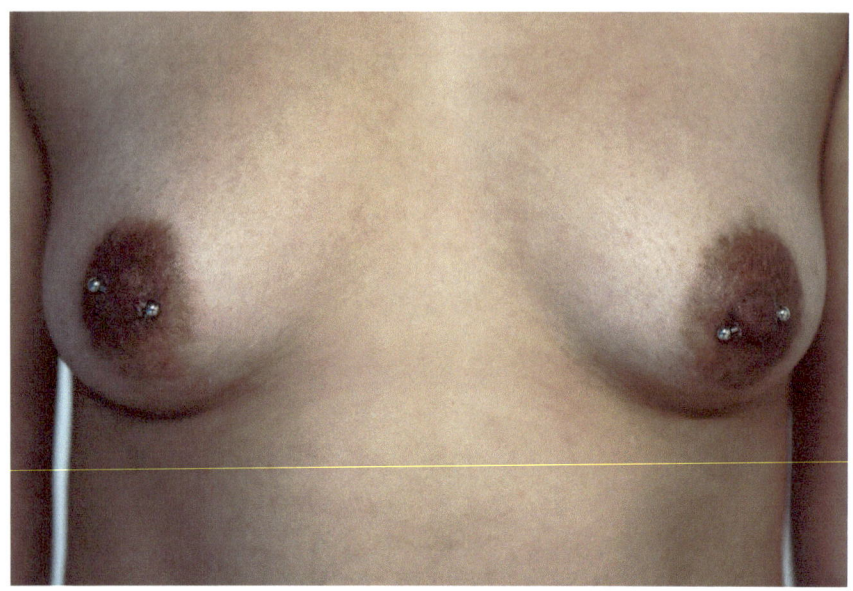

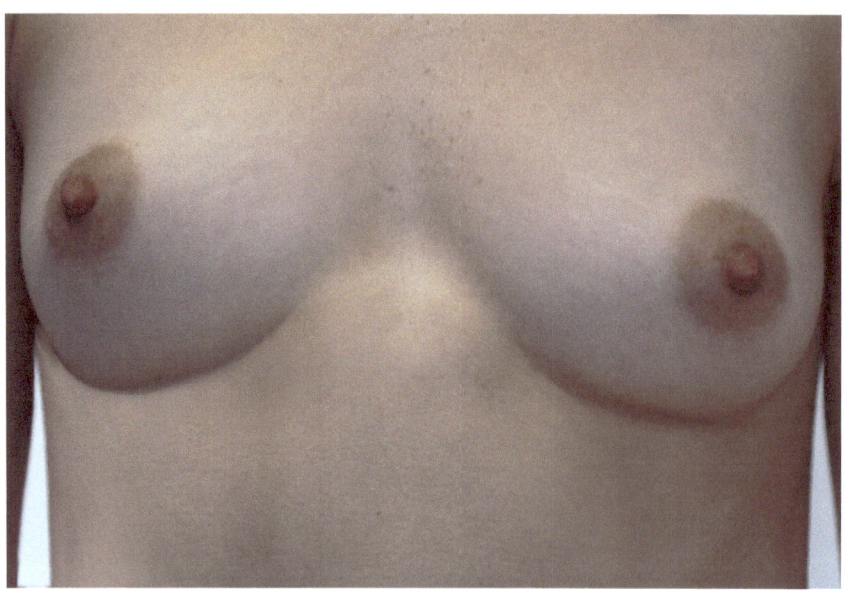

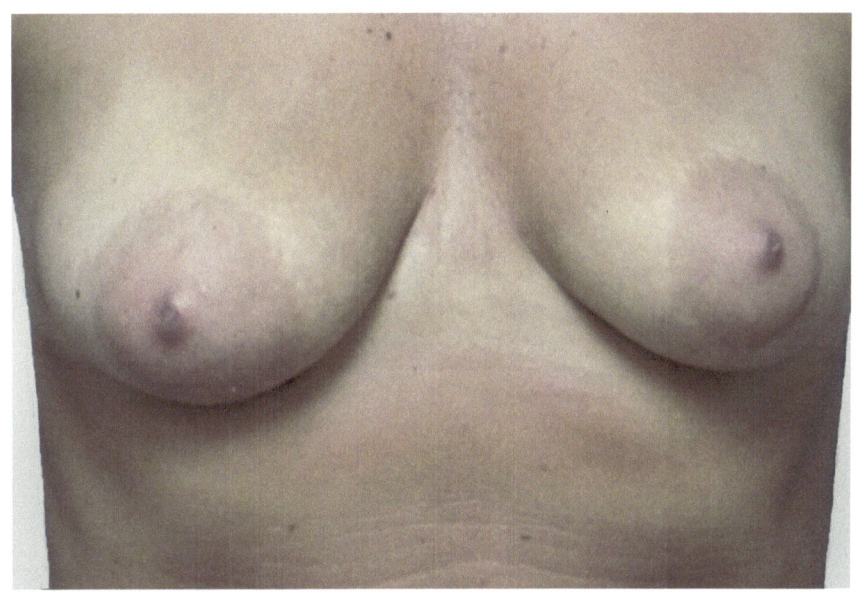

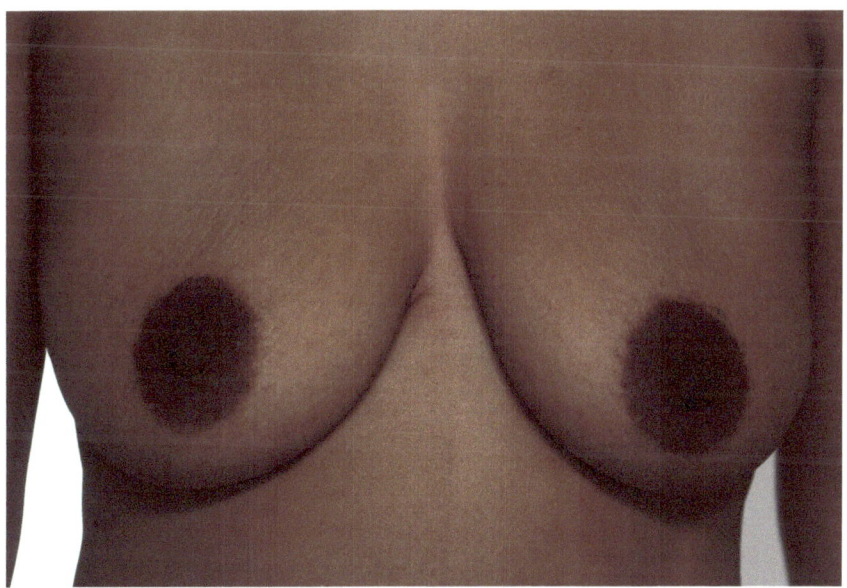

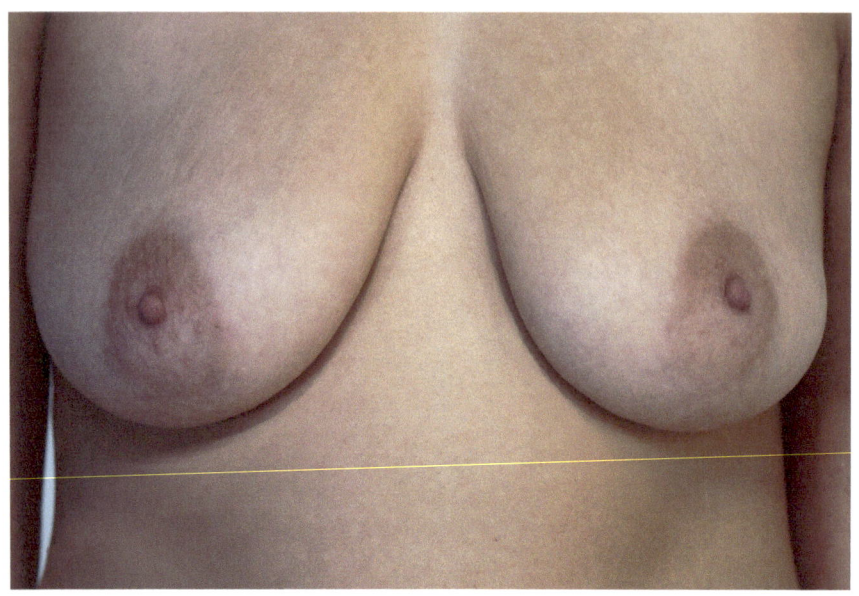

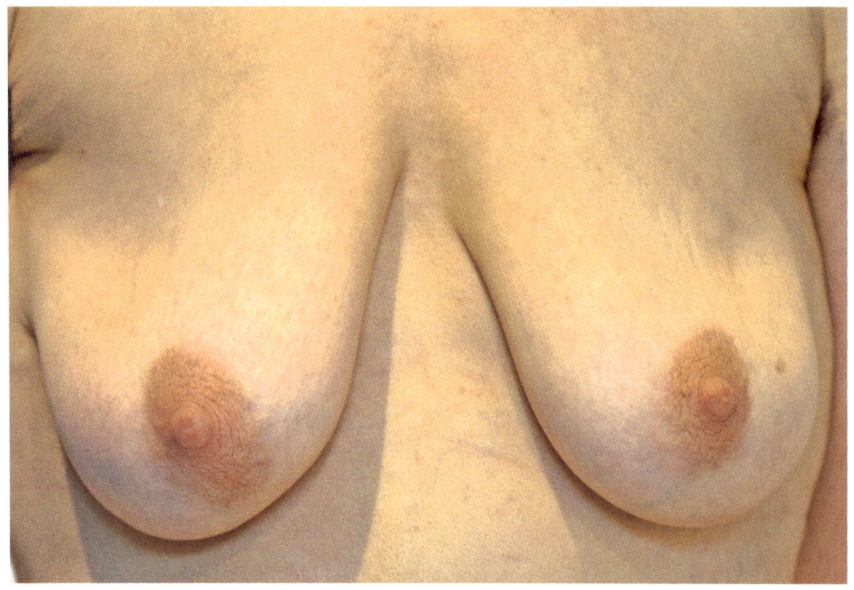

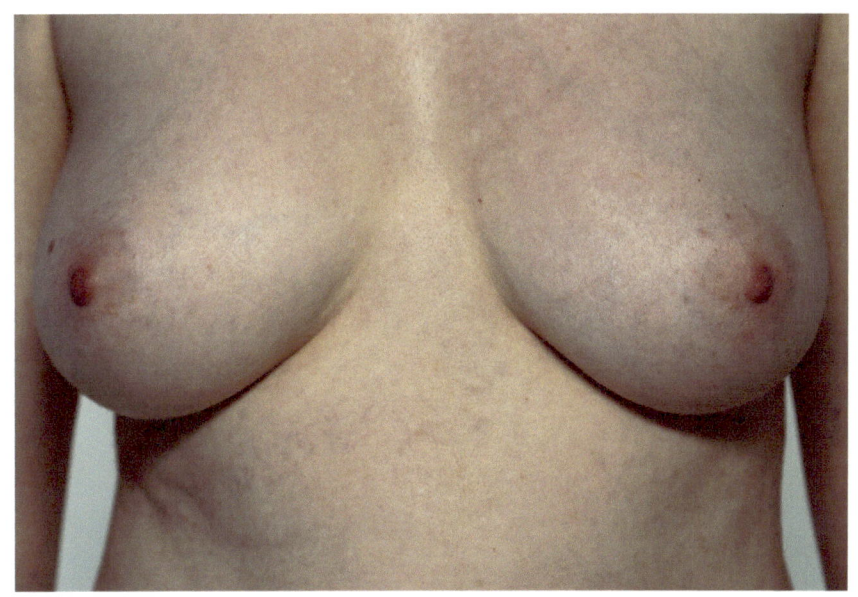

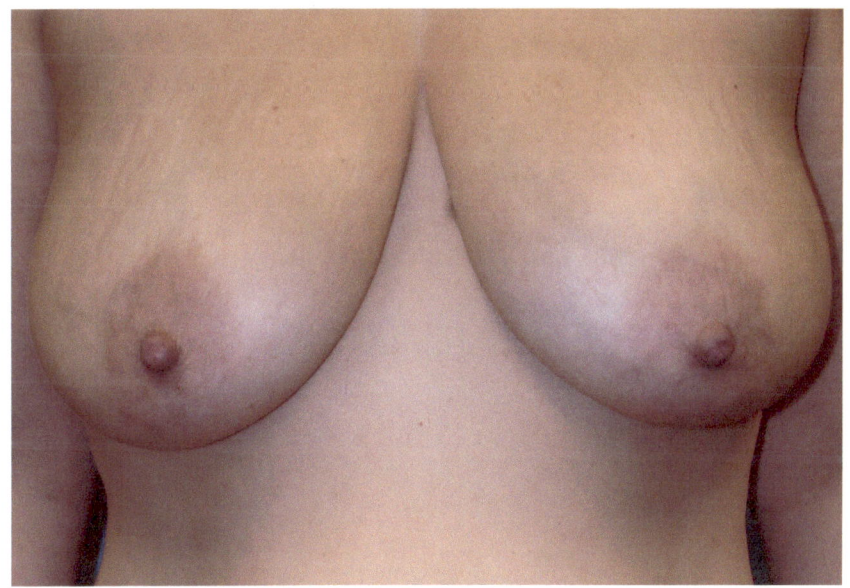

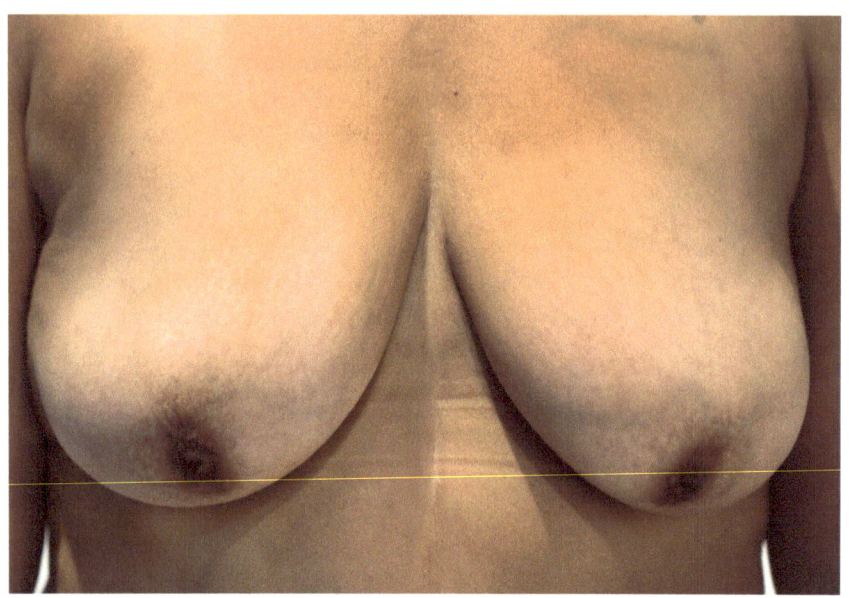

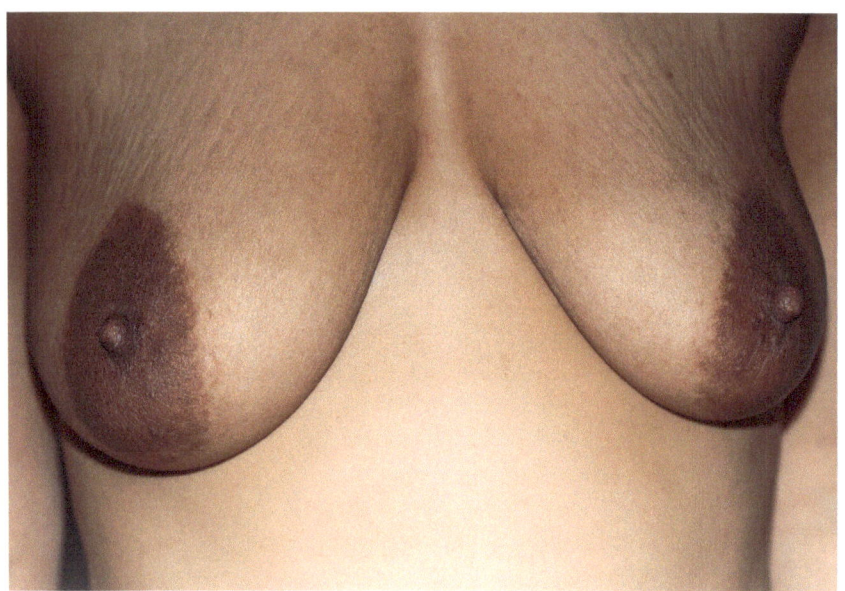

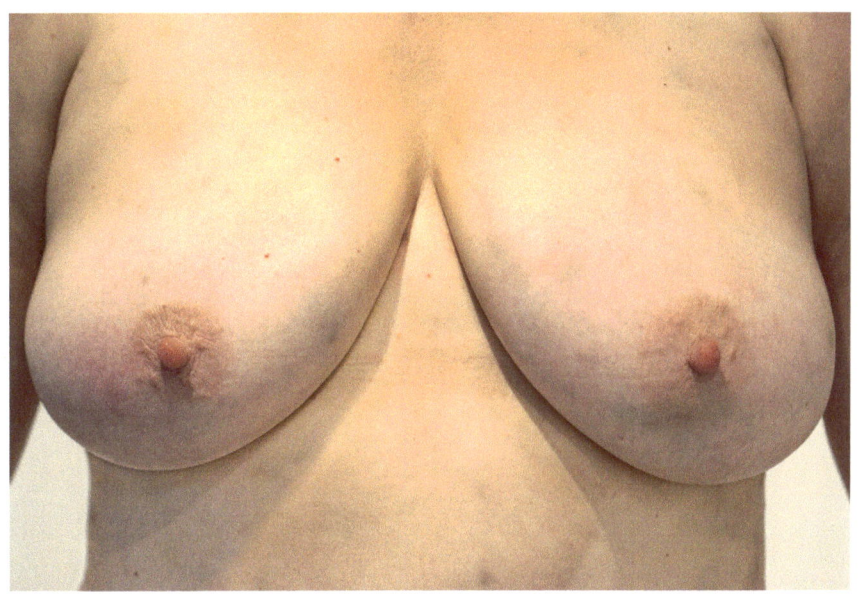

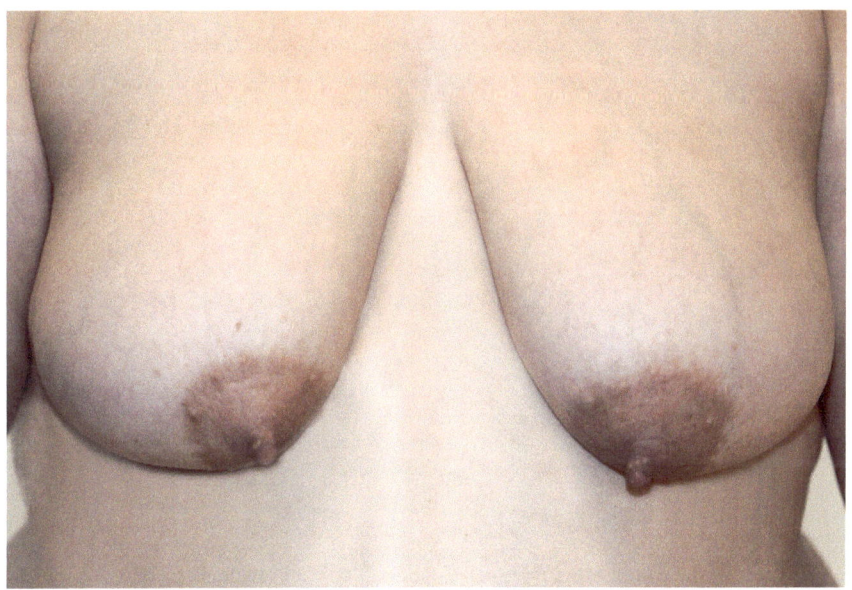

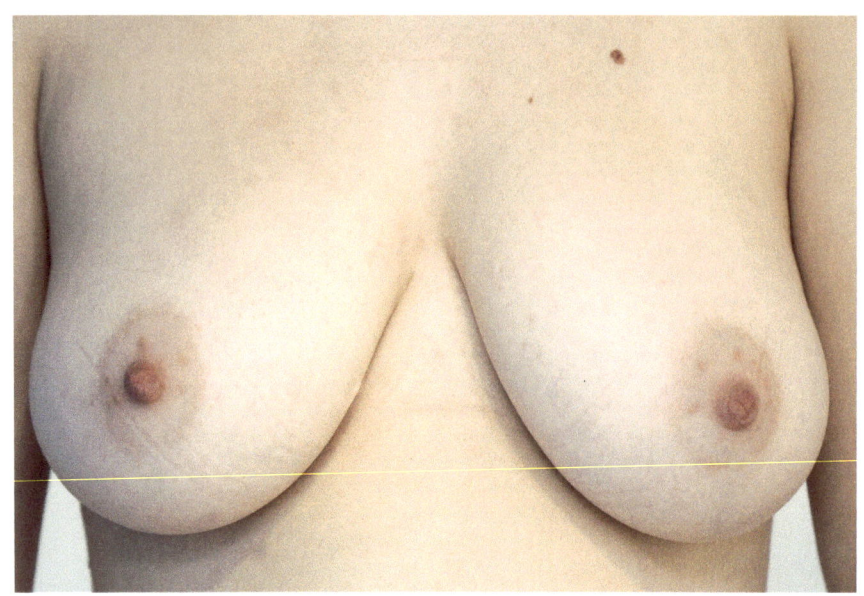

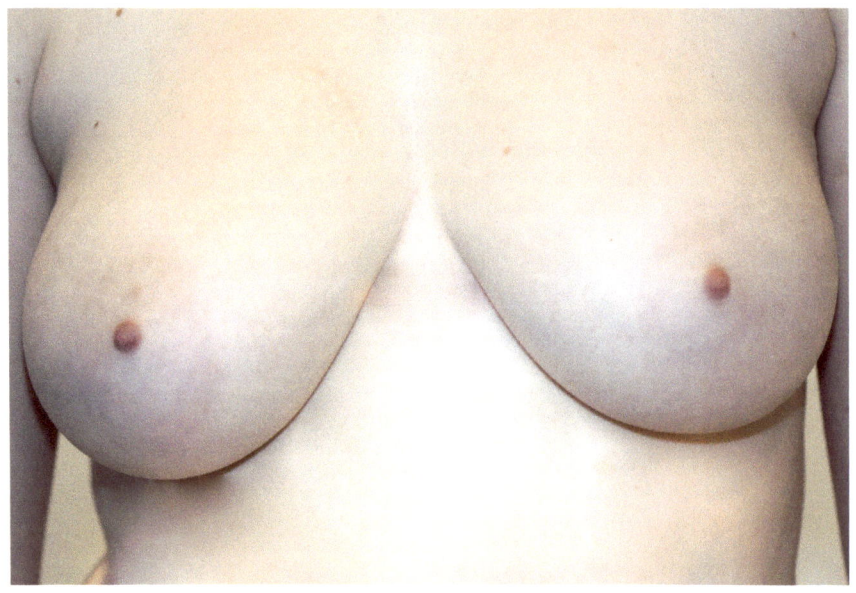

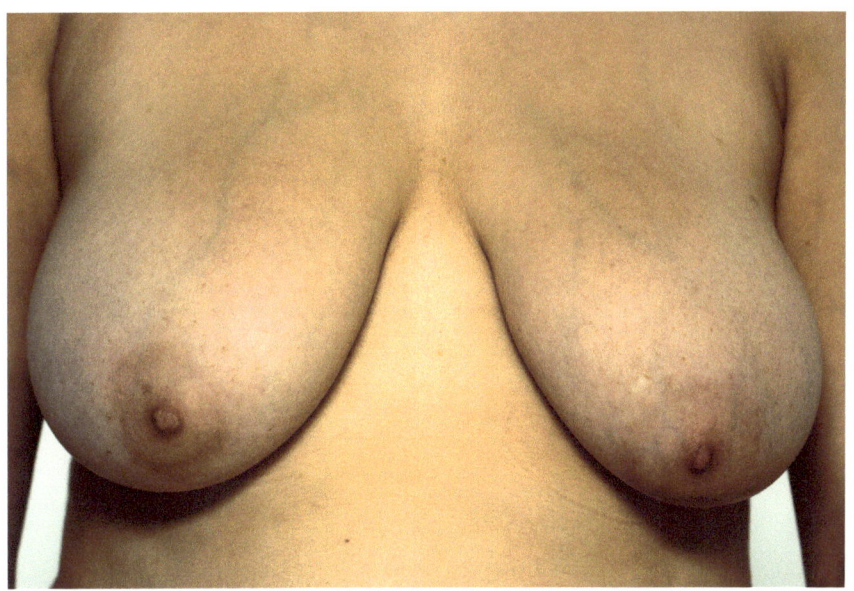

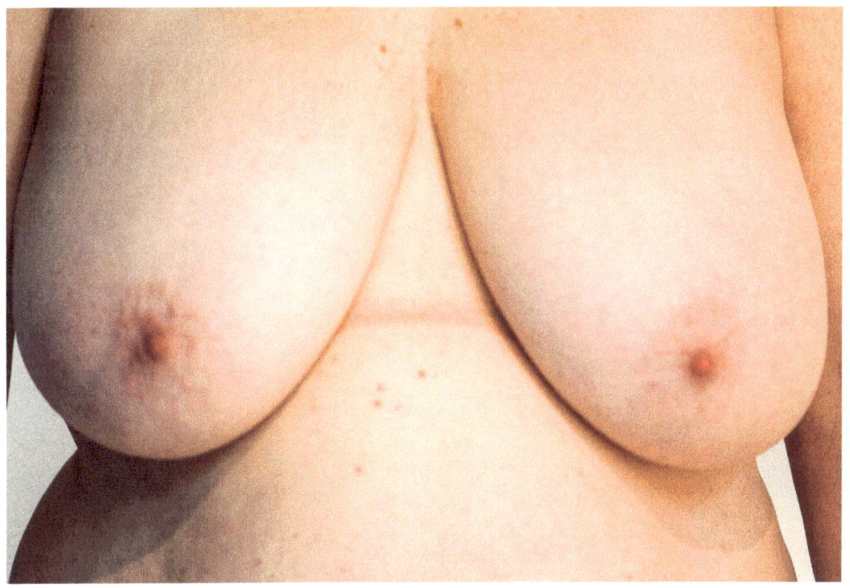

The Breast

The breast refers to the chest area of the body. In humans the breasts refer to a woman's mammary glands, designed specifically to produce milk to feed our young.

Breasts are largely fatty and connective tissue with glands called lobules and ductal (tube-like) structures that, when stimulated by pregnancy and birthing hormones, produce and distribute milk. At the tip of the breasts is the nipple, surrounded by a colored area known as the areola.

Breasts are as individual as women are; their look and anatomy changes as the female body ages.

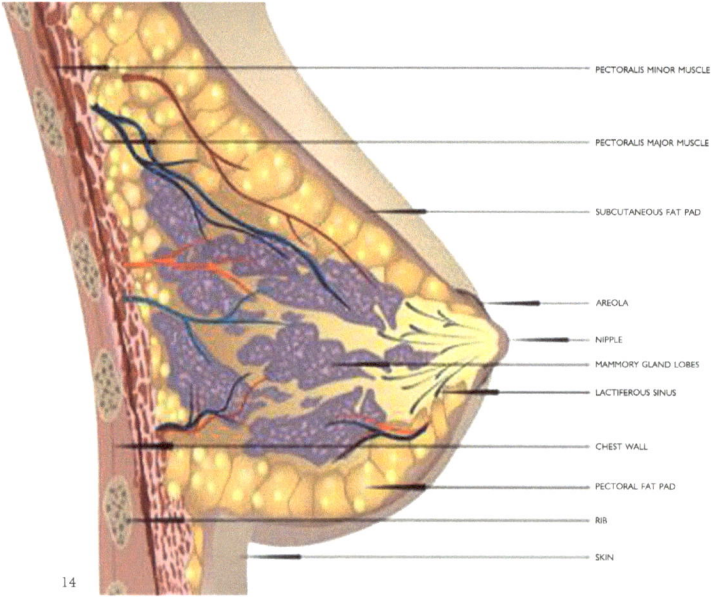

PECTORALIS MINOR MUSCLE

PECTORALIS MAJOR MUSCLE

SUBCUTANEOUS FAT PAD

AREOLA

NIPPLE

MAMMORY GLAND LOBES

LACTIFEROUS SINUS

CHEST WALL

PECTORAL FAT PAD

RIB

SKIN

14

They Are Not Just Accessories, People!

Thus far, this book has focused on what we see. As much as the breasts represent femininity and sexuality, what they really are is a feeding machine. The mammalian breast is the organ used to nourish a species' young. It's a fact: breasts are designed to feed our babies.

It is also a fact that breast milk produces the best nourishment for infants, including the provision of natural immunity directly from their mothers. According to the American Academy of Pediatrics in their 2012 Policy Statement on Breastfeeding, exclusively breast-fed infants have greater protection from ear infections, colds, and digestive problems, as well as fewer incidences of allergies and skin disorders. In their first year of life, the incidence of SIDS (Sudden Infant Death Syndrome) is one-third lower for breast-fed infants. Longer term, there is proof that breastfed infants will have 15-30% less chance of adolescent or adult obesity.[15] The AAP recommends "exclusive breastfeeding for about the first six months of a baby's life, followed by breastfeeding in combination with the introduction of complementary foods until at least 12 months of age, and continuation of breastfeeding for as long as mutually desired by mother and baby." The World Health Organization and UNICEF agree, though they endorse breastfeeding until 2 years of age.

In the United States, an average of 80% of mothers will breastfeed their newborn; almost 50% are still breastfeeding when the infant reaches six months-old, and half that many continue through the baby's first birthday. Interestingly, the rate of breastfeeding is not tied to how populated a state is, but there are regional trends. More women choose to breastfeed and continue for a longer duration in the Rocky Mountain and Pacific areas than women in the Mid-Atlantic, South and Southwest.[16]

The numbers of women who choose to breastfeed varies around the world. It is lowest in South Asia and Sub-Saharan Africa, so much so that as few as 39% of infants are introduced to breastfeeding within an hour of birth. This number matters because non-breastfed infants have more than a 40% prevalence of stunted growth and 14x greater likelihood of early childhood death from diarrhea or pneumonia.[17] An increase in the rate and duration of breastfeeding has the potential to prevent over hundreds of thousands of deaths (13% of all deaths) in children under five in the developing world.[18]

The WHO, UNICEF and countless government health agencies have initiatives in place to increase breastfeeding rates among all women. Exclusively breastfeeding infants for six months and continuing to breastfeed while adding appropriate starter foods for infants under two years of age has a higher impact on child survival than any other health intervention. More importantly, good childhood nutrition has long-term consequences for better health that in turn has a positive impact on children's cognitive ability. The potential for improved health and learning can potentially impact economic productivity and provide a chance to break the cycle of poverty and illness that has stymied these underdeveloped countries for generations.[18]

In 1992, the WHO and UNICEF launched the Baby-Friendly Hospital Initiative (BFHI) which since has been adopted by more than 16,000 hospitals in 171 countries worldwide. BFHI provides an inpatient support system that has enabled more than seven out of ten women to initiate breastfeeding upon delivery. For many families in need, lactation support is not readily available once a woman takes her baby home and the percentage of infants being fed breast milk drops significantly after a month and precipitously after three months. Following on the success of BFHI, the WHO and UNICEF published their Global Strategy for Infant and Young Child Feeding in 2005. Their objectives are to continue raising awareness of infant and child nutrition, to impress upon governments and international organizations the importance of establishing legal and support mechanisms for breastfeeding mothers, their infants and young children and to ask for adoption of the International Code of Marketing Breast Milk Substitutes.

Breastfeeding is beneficial to mothers as well as babies. For mothers, breastfeeding helps limit maternal post-delivery bleeding, it has been linked to a reduced incidence of post-partum depression,[19] and it facilitates the female body returning to its pre-pregnancy state. Longer term, there is evidence that breastfeeding reduces the rate of Type 2 Diabetes, and breast, uterine and ovarian cancers.[20] Best of all is the practicality of nursing – breast milk is there when you need it, sterile, warm and free.

There is widespread agreement that breast milk is the ideal diet for infants. Yet controversy has arisen, especially in urban areas of the United States, about the delivery system used to provide this optimal nourishment. People opposed to public breastfeeding claim it is "indecent exposure," "awkward," "too sexual" and have arguments to back their case. Supporters counter with equally reasonable assertions. The more restrictive the state legislation, the lower the rate of breastfeeding in that state.[21]

Between nursing bras, a woman's clothing and the baby, other than seeing a bit more skin than usual, the breast is blocked from view. Be sensitive to those around you. If you are uncomfortable with a woman breastfeeding in public then do not look. And ladies, understand that there may be someone who feels awkward seeing a woman nurse their baby. So try to be discreet – it is possible to breastfeed a baby so that no one sees anything more than a baby cuddled to your chest and perhaps some décolletage. Mutual courtesy is not very difficult.

In developed countries with sanitary water supplies, there are healthy alternatives for women who physically cannot breastfeed, or who choose not to nurse their infants. Babies fed store-bought, government health authority or medically approved, infant formulas will get 100% of their nutritional requirements met and there are countless ways to provide closeness, nurturing and love.

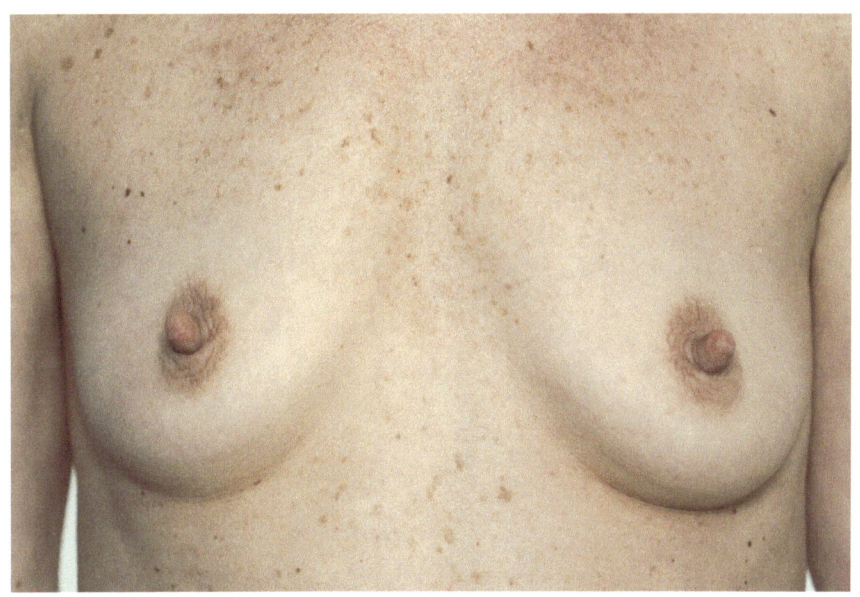

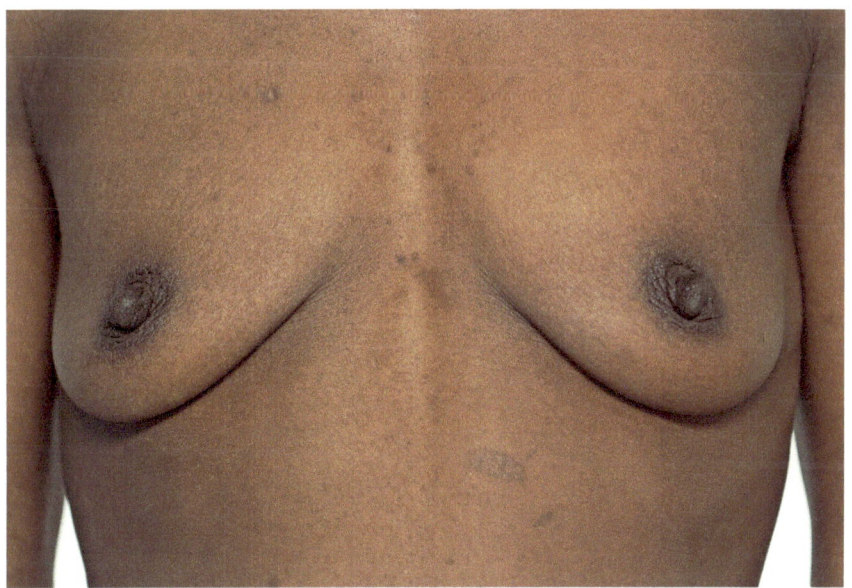

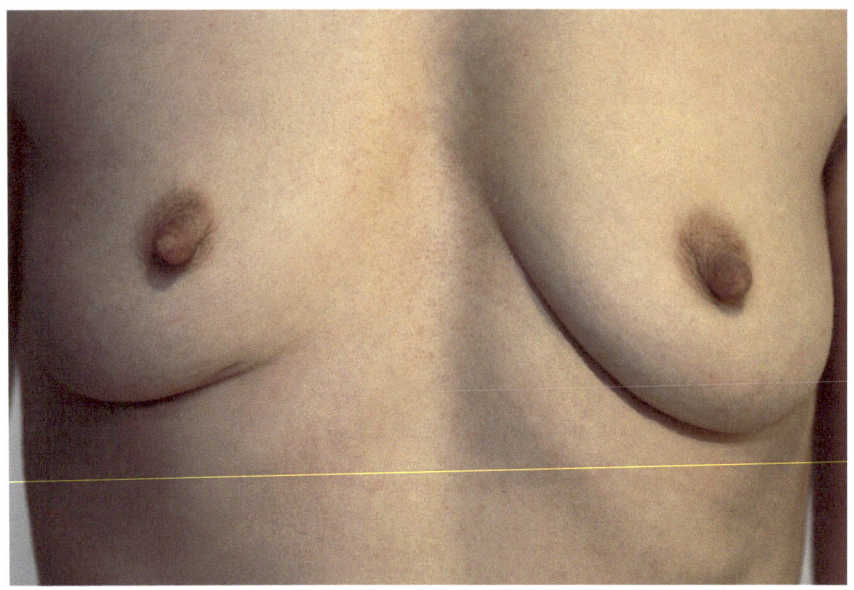

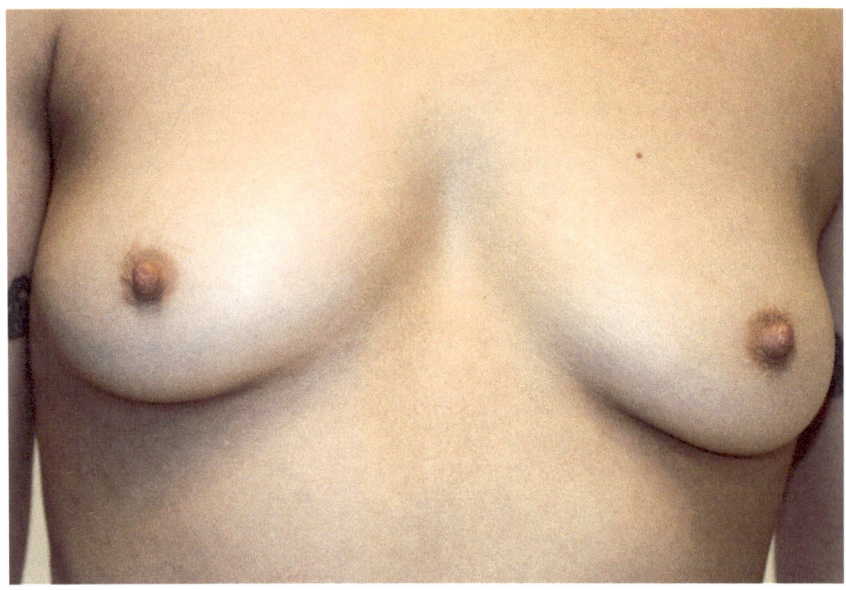

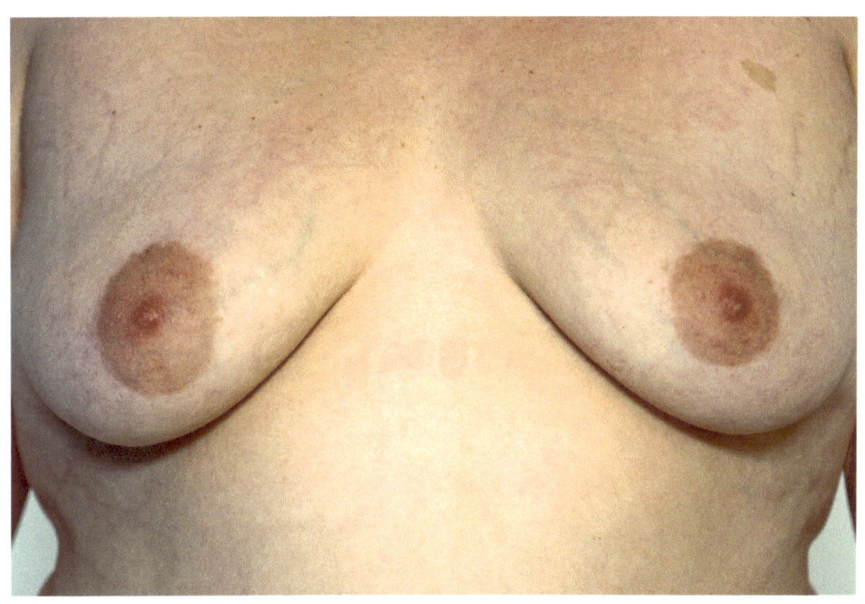

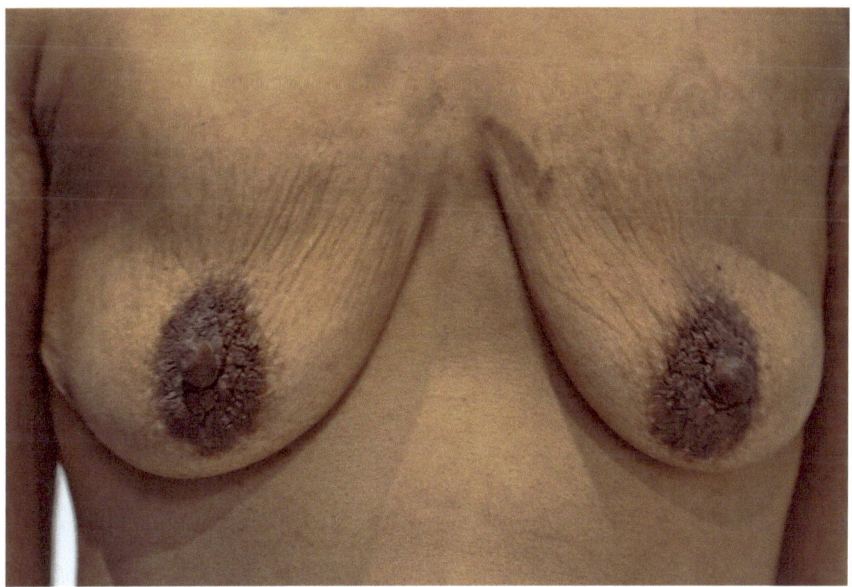

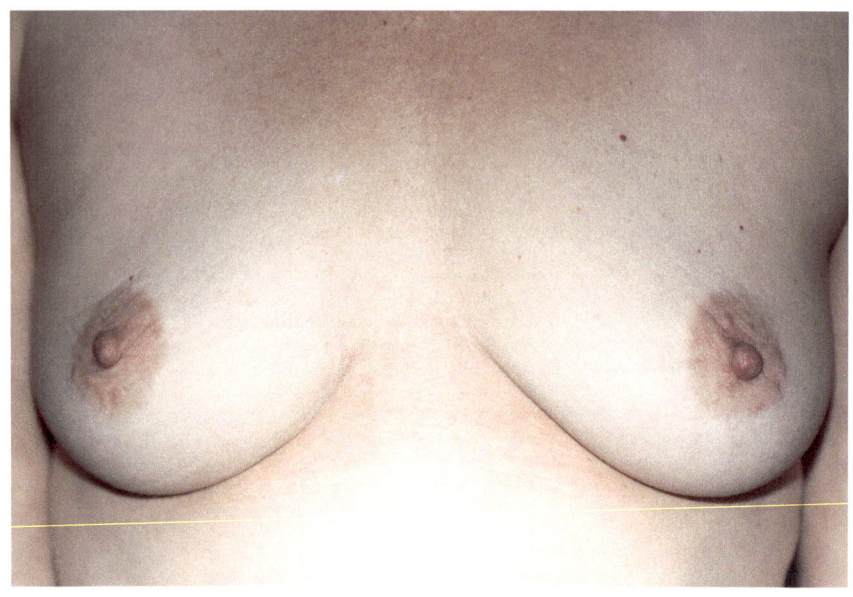

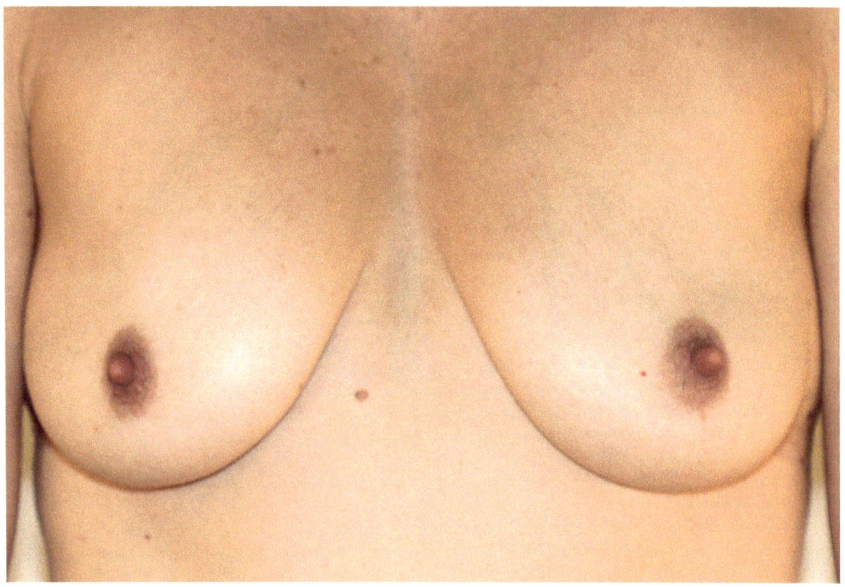

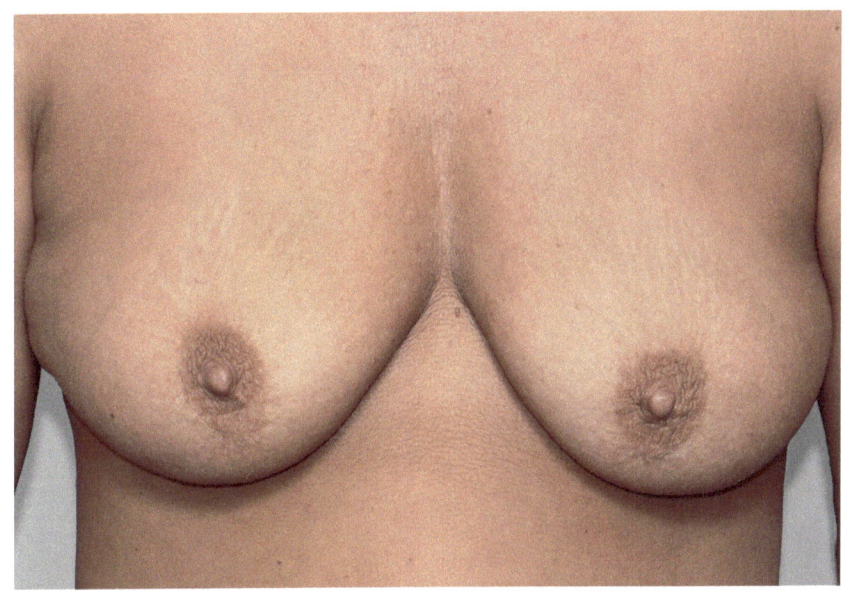

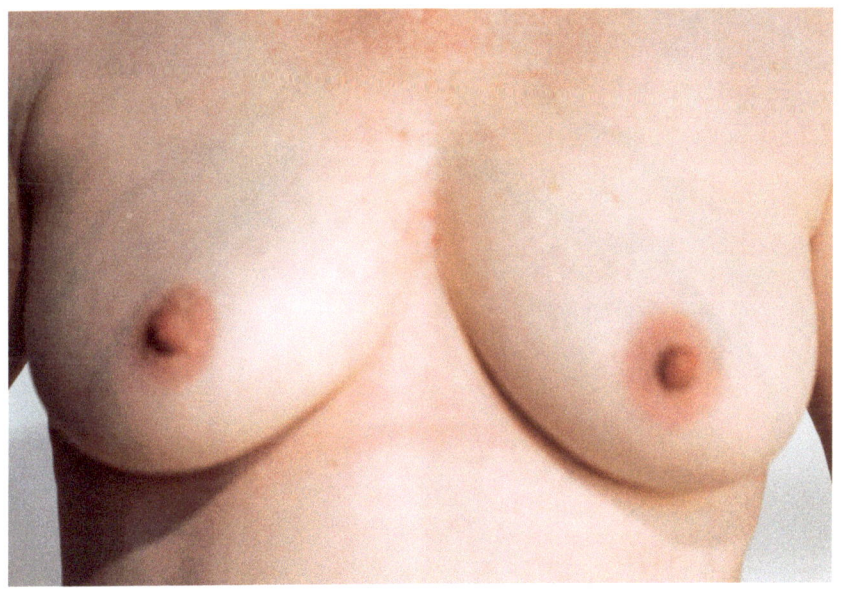

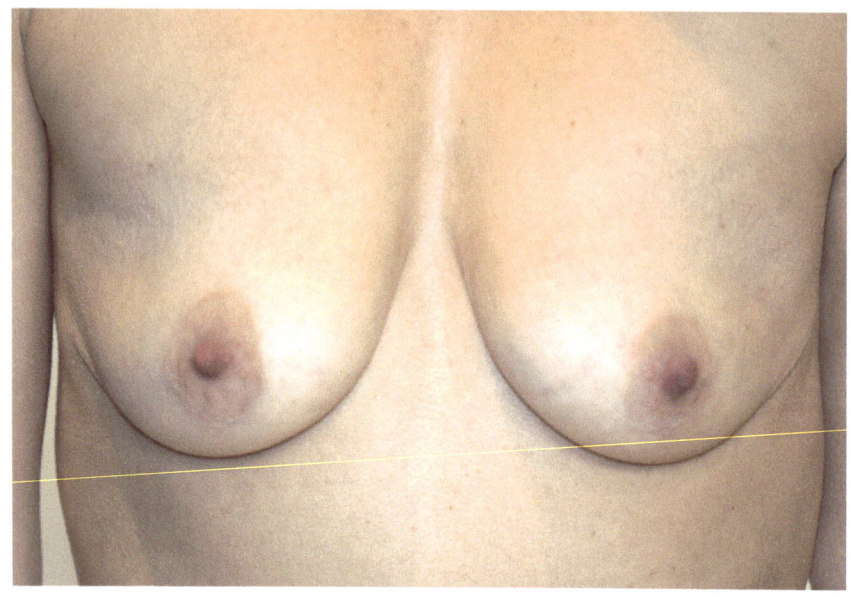

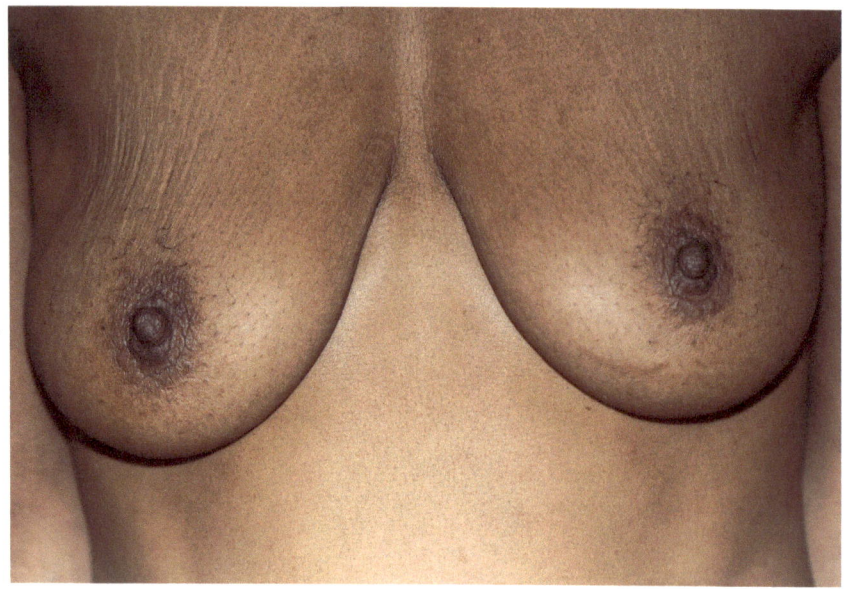

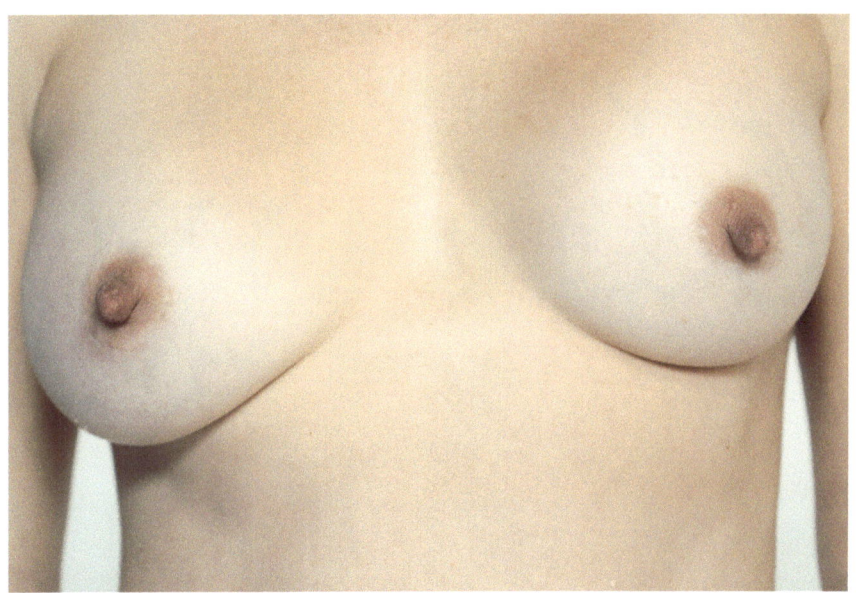

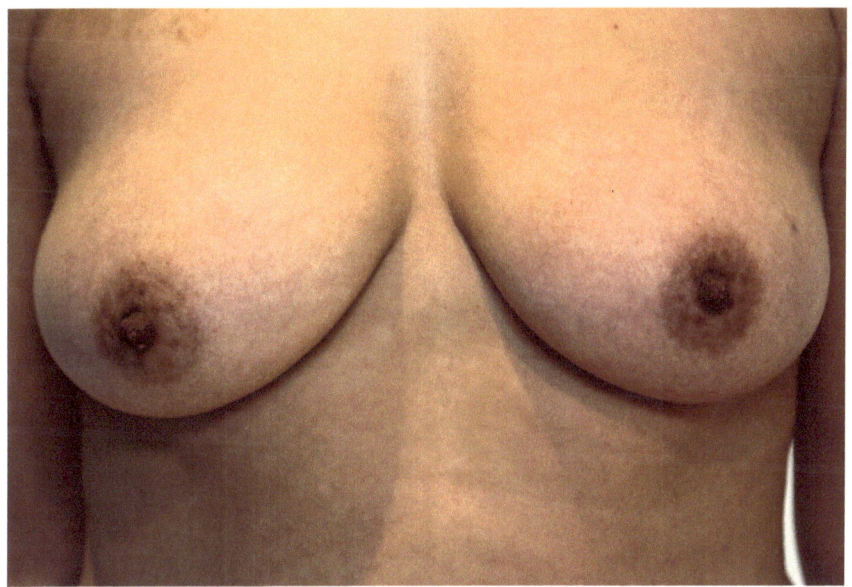

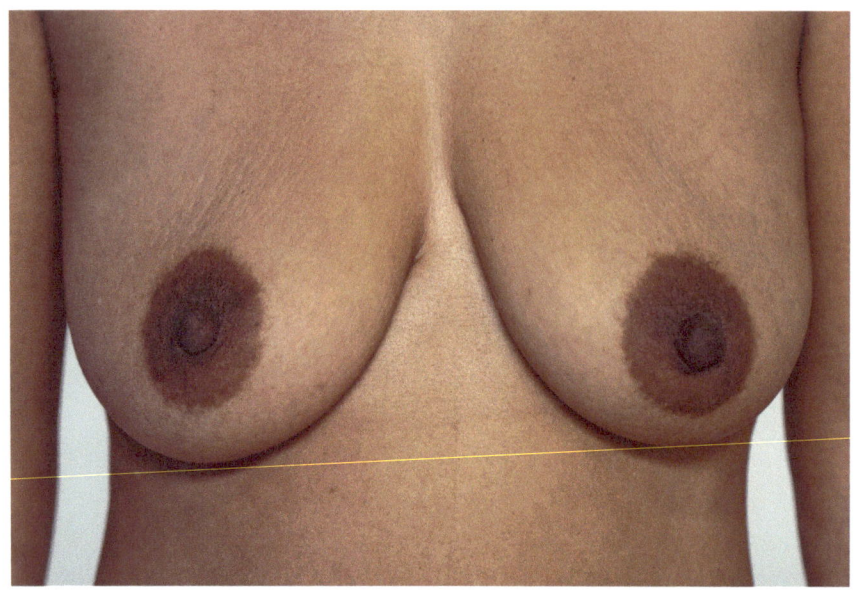

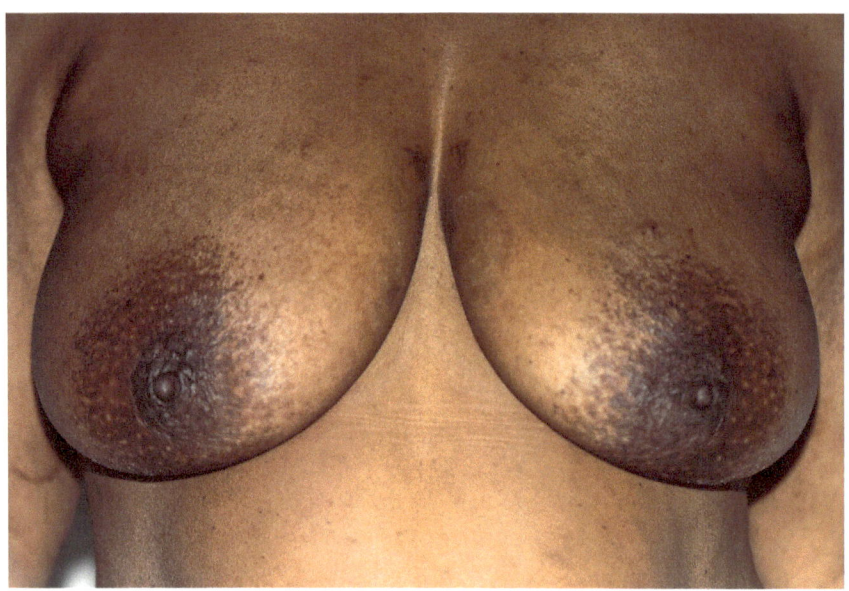

Who Are These Women? <small>continued</small>

There was a group of women familiar with my first publication, *The Private Square Volume 1: Penises,* who contacted me via the TPS website asking to participate in my research. Graduate students in a nearby university's Sexuality Studies program impressed me with their deep-seated belief that no one should be objectified for their body. If most young adults were as accepting of all people regardless of their looks or sexuality, our society will change for the better. Two of them wanted to pursue a career in academia. Another, who had spent time as a Peace Corp volunteer and later an ESL teacher, wanted to use her experience and education in the public policy arena. Meeting them reaffirmed my conviction that change occurs one person and one step at a time. Thank you ladies.

A woman nearing seventy had much to say in general about breasts. It was clear that with her years came much perspective and wisdom. Among her senior crowd, she claimed the attitude of women with smaller breasts was "Breasts? Who cares?". Her friends with larger breasts thought they were more a nuisance that anything else. All wanted to have command of their own bodies – her friends who had experienced breast cancer treatment and surgery universally felt they lost that control to the disease.

An early client contacted me months after her photo shoot. A woman in her late forties, she had lost 30 pounds and wanted to know if I could retake her pictures. I agreed. Two other women I photographed had lost even more weight – about 100 pounds each. Since much of the breast is adipose tissue, aka fat, changes in weight have a visible affect. The younger, healthier and more physically fit a person is, the more elasticity their skin has to adjust a smaller body.

Included among my photo subjects were three women who worked as Life Figure Models. Unlike entertainment industry representatives, these women were not 5'8" to 5'10" tall, weighing less than 125 and wearing size 00-2. They could be you, your sister, your mother, or your friend.

One mused that only in recent history has thinness been associated with women's beauty – art history through the ages show curviness as one of the standards of femininity.

Another was in a leadership position with a local Life Figure Model association and shared that virtually all of their members, women and men alike, did not fit the fashion model mode.

The third life model was an artist who, after decades of identifying herself as a painter, decided she could make art via modeling instead. Life Figure Model gigs allowed her to demonstrate to students of all ages that beauty is all about how individuals interpret what they see. This woman shared that scores of students had drawn, painted or sculpted her body. Over the years, though her looks were relatively constant, not a single piece of their art was ever the same.

The handful of models who had their nipples pierced were all Millennials. Regardless of your personal opinion on the practice, and whether you would make that choice yourself, here is a compilation of reasons they gave for making the decision to have the piercing done. These women cautioned others to use a reliable piercer who is licensed, has experience, recommendations (preferably personal referrals), and practices Universal Precautions.

- The piercings are attractive and pretty
- They can increase nipple sensitivity
- Piercings can make your nipples stand out more
- It is a secret piercing; one that only select people get to see
- For the experience
- It is a bit kinky and they show open-mindedness
- They make me feel sexy
- Love the way they feel to touch on my body
- Hope that they add an interesting twist to sexy times

Many of the women and men who had participated in my research were quite generous and freely shared their feelings about women's breasts. Regardless of ethnicity, socio-economic status or education, people in their 20s focus significantly greater attention on breasts. They care more than twice as much as those in their 30s about the overall look – size, shape, nipples – of their own and others' breasts. The majority of women queried agreed that as they passed through the decades of their lifecycle, breasts become less sexualized, more utilitarian and ultimately, outside of health issues, not a concern.

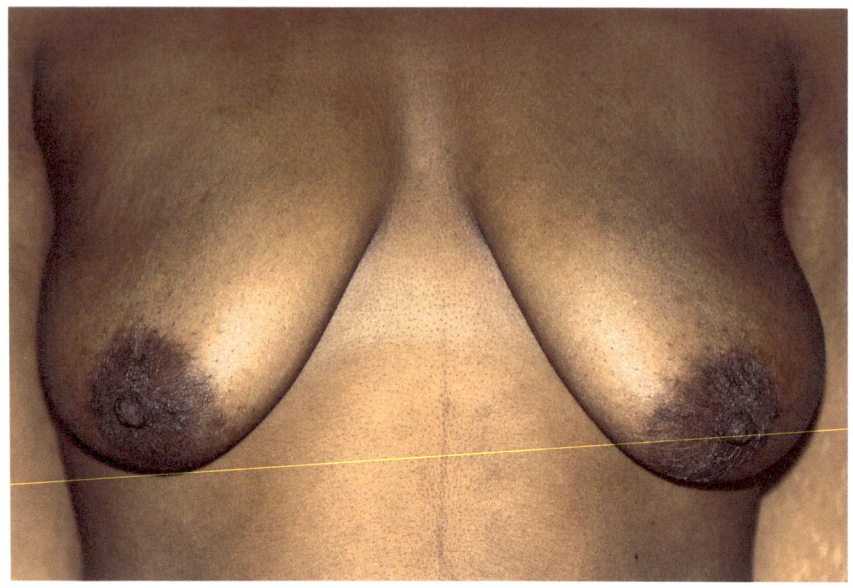

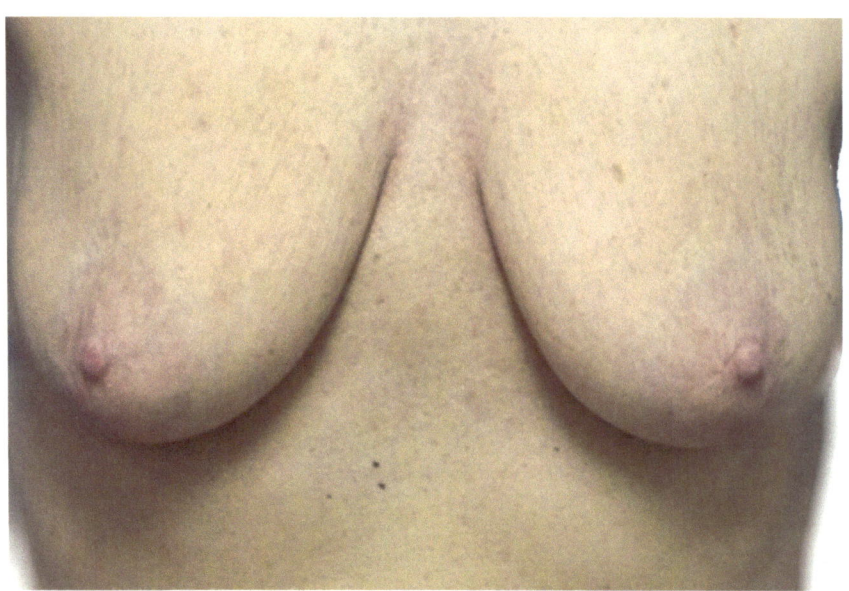

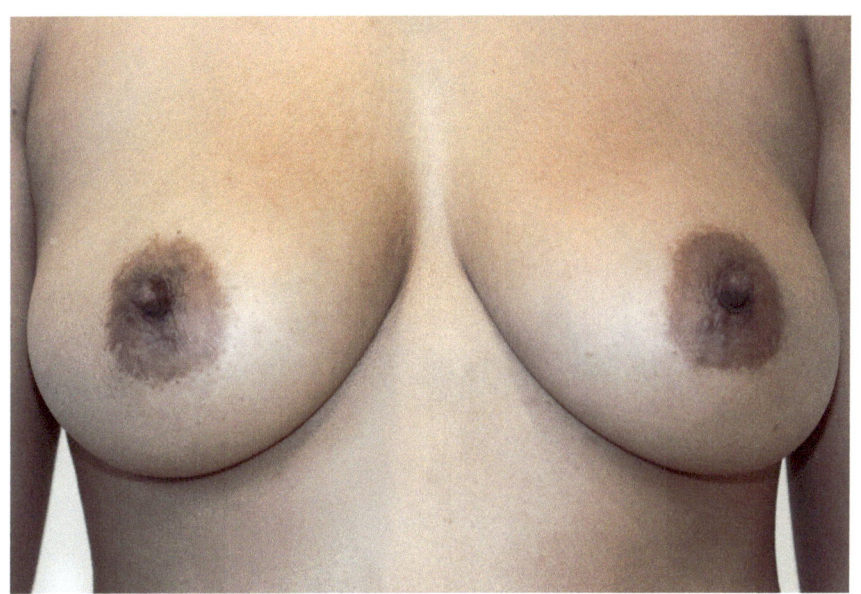

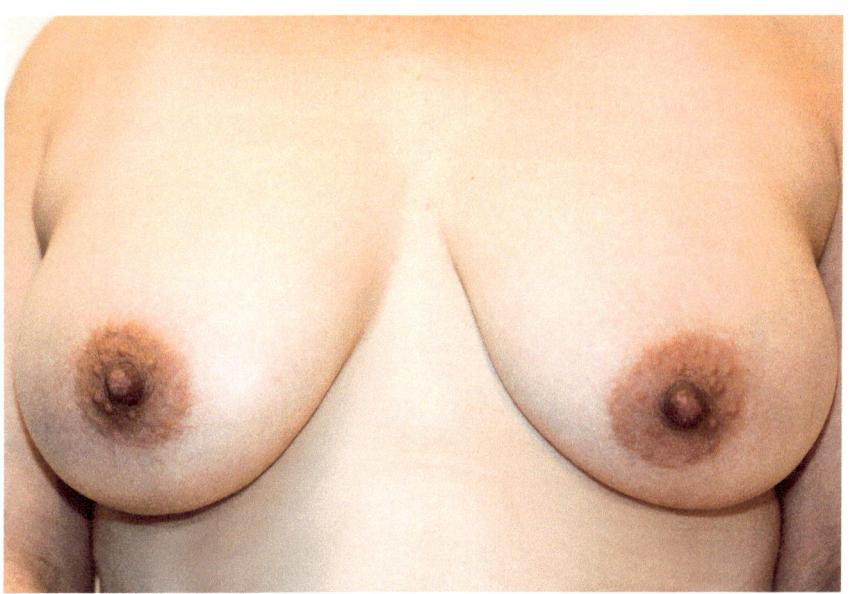

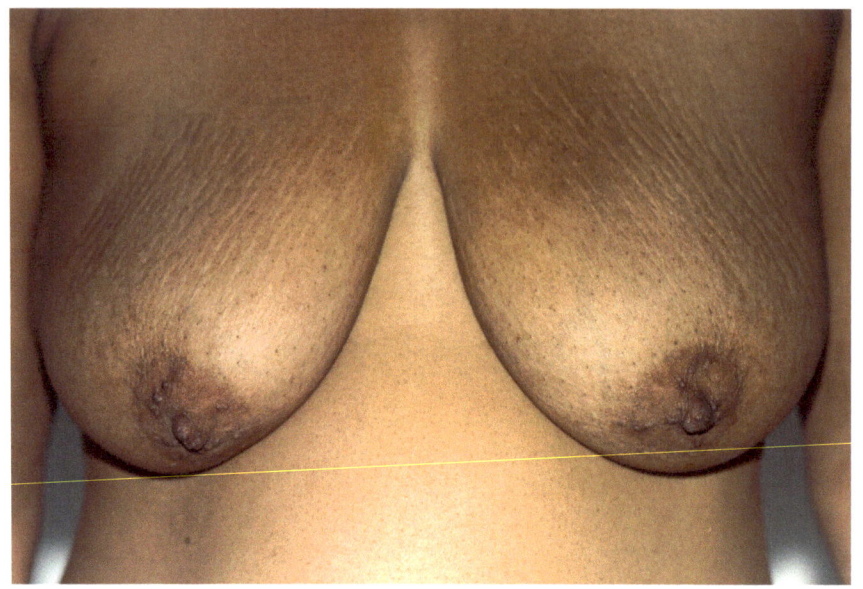

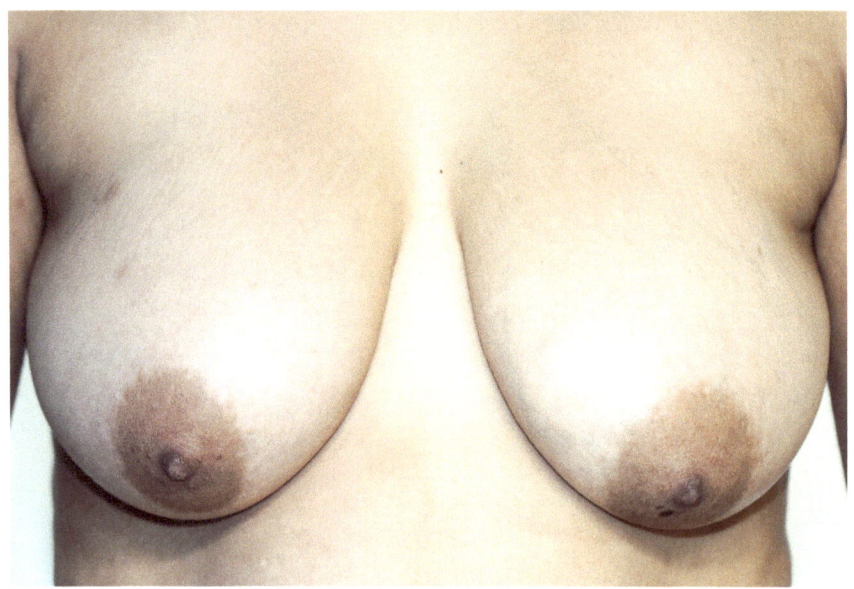

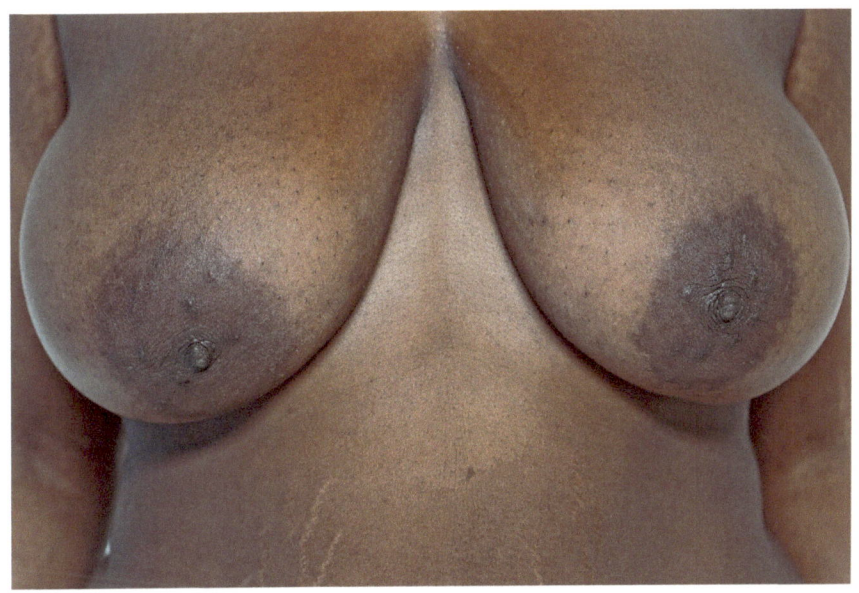

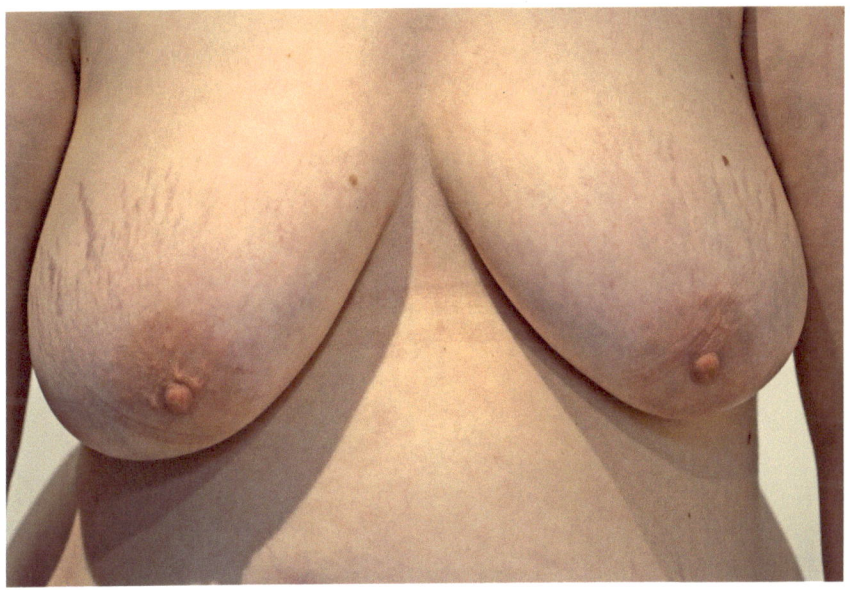

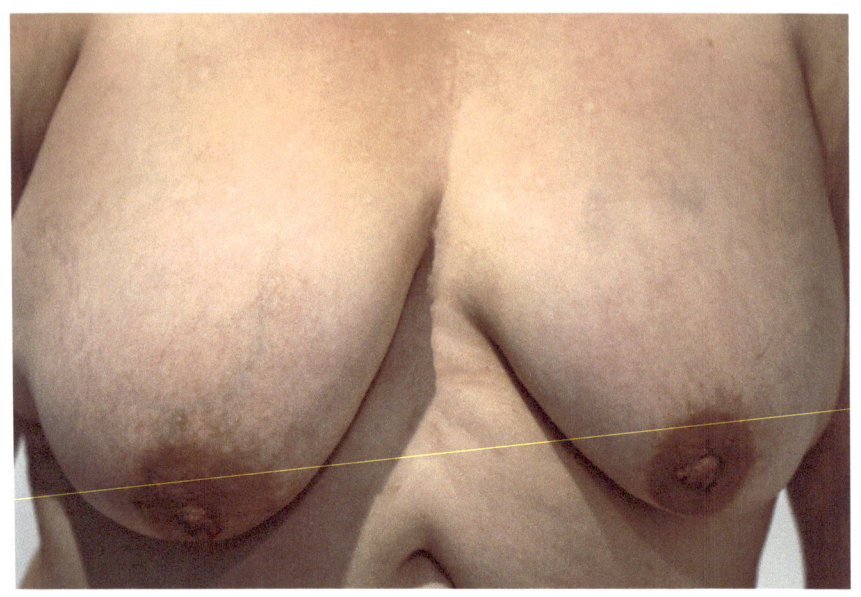

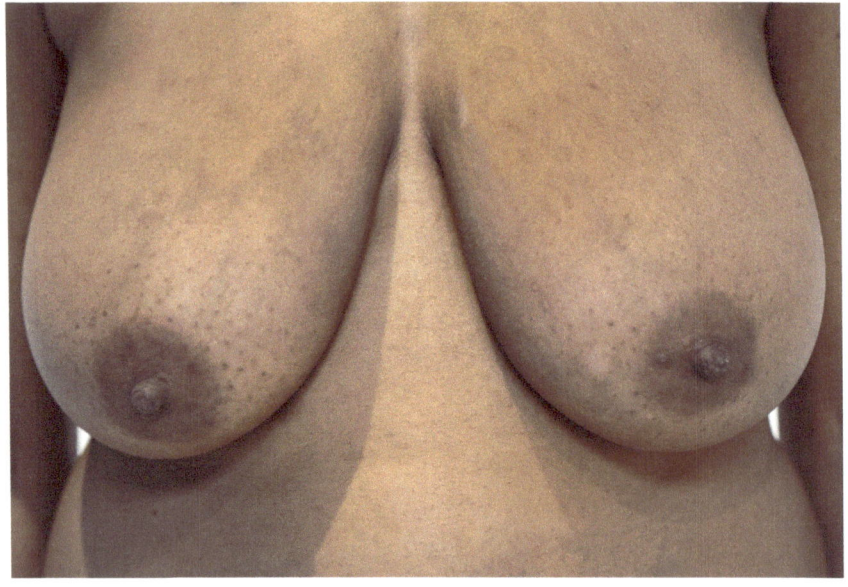

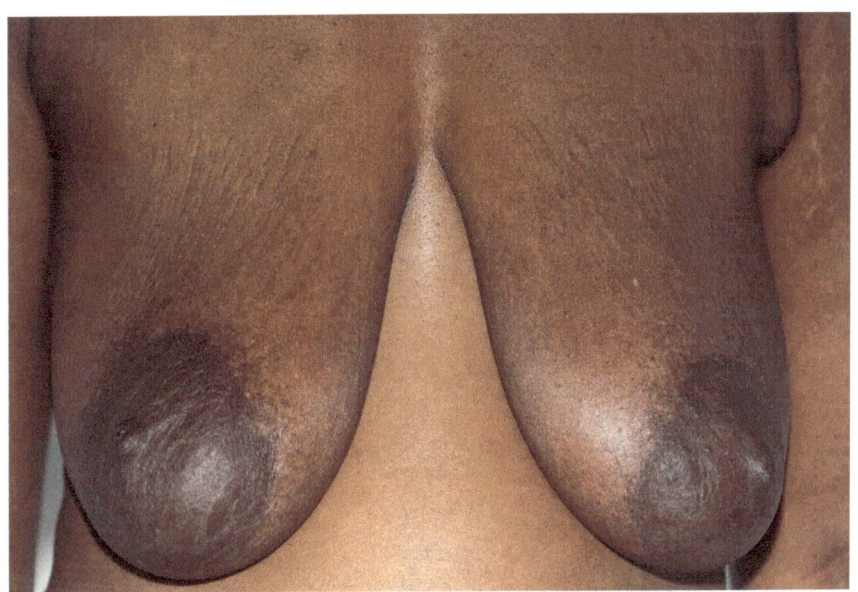

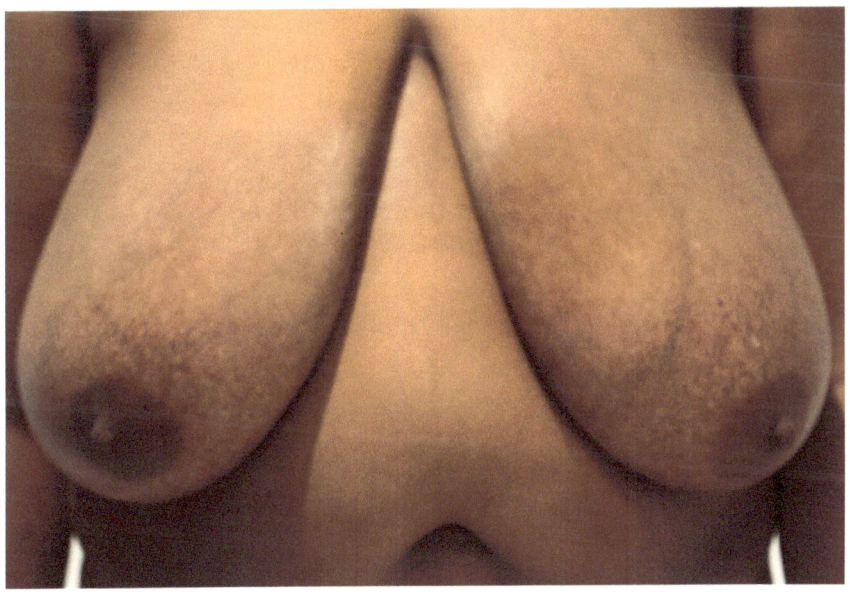

OBJECTIFICATION & SEXUALIZATION

Millions of women in major, industrialized nations are seeking a more perfect pair of breasts. Since the advent of the big screen and the Barbie™ doll, what constitutes feminine beauty has narrowed. Though there are examples of photo manipulation as early as an iconic 1860 portrait of Abraham Lincoln (it was Lincoln's head affixed on Southern politician John Calhoun's body), one of the earliest examples of using the technique to alter a photograph to improve a woman's figure may be TV Guide's August 1989 cover of Oprah Winfrey's head on Ann-Margret's body, modified without either woman's permission.[22] Countless times since then, fashion and social magazines especially have digitally altered featured photographs to enhance breasts, slim waists and legs, smooth hips, round buttocks, enlarge muscles and more. Not until GQ published a noticeably slender version of Kate Winslet on the January 2003 cover, did someone speak out. In a nationally aired complaint, Winslet said that the retouching was "excessive." She continued, saying: "I don't look like that and more importantly I don't desire to look like that. I can tell you that they've reduced the size of my legs by about a third."[21] Not only does Kate Winslet not look as depicted, neither does virtually any model, male or female who grace the pages of these publications. What has been propagated as part of the ultimate female body – breasts that are symmetric, round, full, high and perky, with perfectly sized areolae and nipples projected just-right – is NOT what women's breasts really look like.

According to the American Psychological Association (APA), sexualization can show up in four forms: 1) when a person's worth is assumed to only come from his or her sexiness; 2) when a child is expected or encouraged to act or dress sexually; 3) when a person is treated as a sex object rather than as a whole person; and/or 4) when physical characteristics are considered to be the only indicator of sexiness. Both females and males can be victims of sexualization.

In August 2011, the University of Buffalo Sociology Department released a study measuring the increasing sexualization in the past few decades of women in the media comparing the covers of Rolling Stones Magazine from 1967 - 2009. In the 1960's, research revealed that 11% of men and 44% of women on the covers of Rolling Stone were sexualized; by the 2000's, these numbers increased to 17% of men and 83% of women being sexualized.[23] For the past fifty years, the post baby-boom population has distorted the free love movement of their teen years into a disrespectful spectacle objectifying women.

In the early 21st century, however, there is chatter in the cloud about changing the focus of body image from conformity to a photo-enhanced or surgically altered figure to that of individual and personal health. I think we have electronic publishing to thank for initiating this welcome and long-overdue change in the media's portrayal of women.

On July 4, 1971 a man named Michael Hart founded the Gutenberg Project to digitize and freely share documents.

In the 1980s the inexpensive, easily shared and transportable compact disk was manufactured and became the means to share vast amounts of information. Cable television proliferated, and those studios deserve a nod for bringing some original programs to us – but their talent still conformed to quite narrow standards of beauty and body image deemed worthy of the screen. In the 1990s eBooks hit the market, followed by advent of ePaper technology in the 2000s that revolutionized the publishing industry opening up authorship to a universe of writers who had previously been denied access. The result is that countless individuals and organizations can air, thus share, information. No longer are a group of entertainment, network or fashion magazine personnel in command of what images and import we are exposed to. Today, however, the shout-out is to the "indie" movement that has captured the attention of the main stream and is showing more and more that beauty comes in all shapes, sizes and colors! As do breasts.

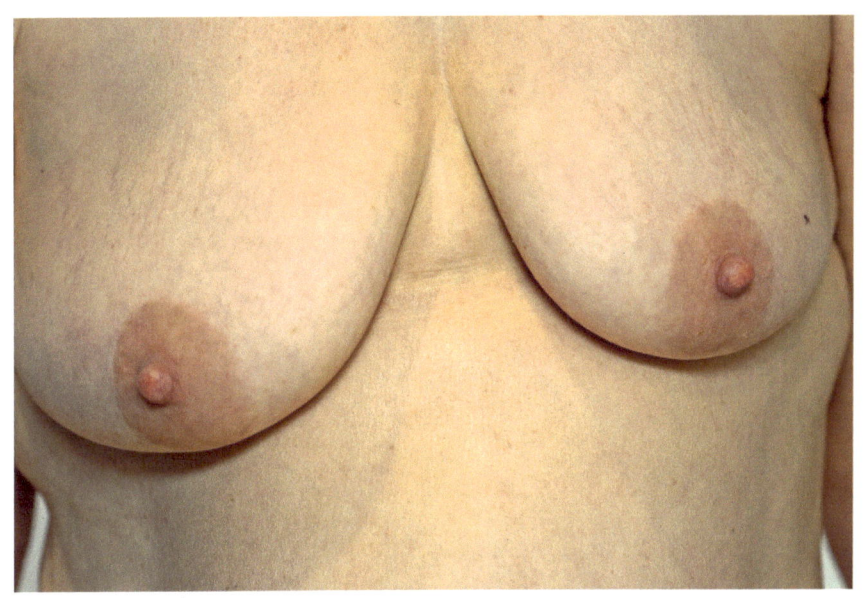

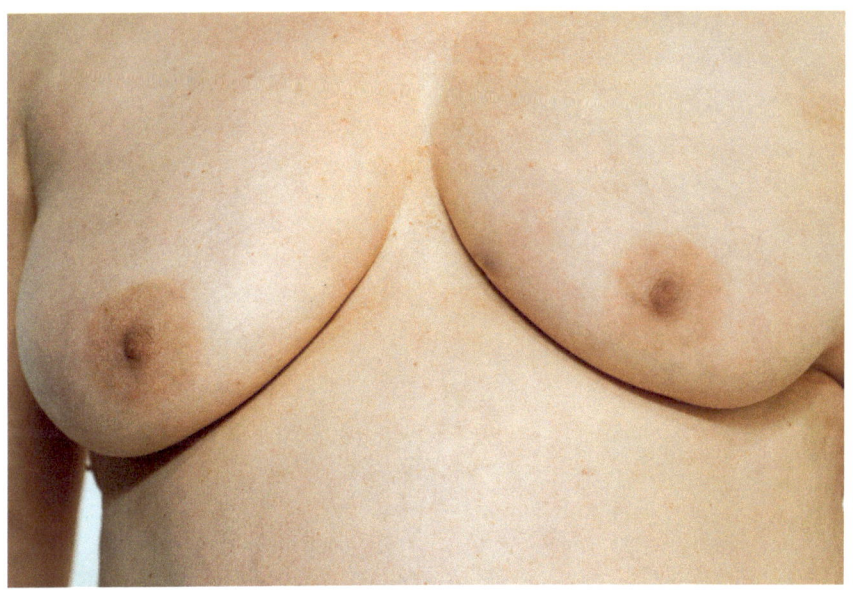

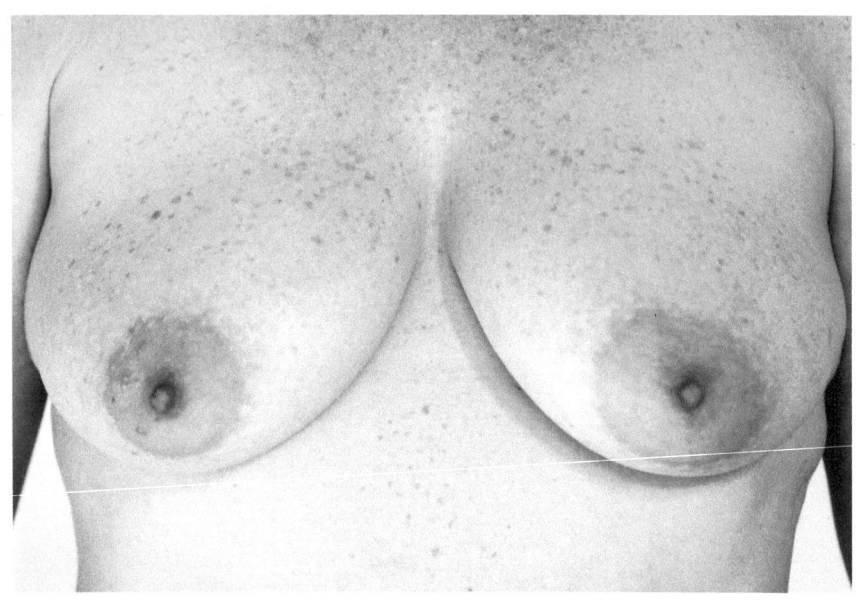

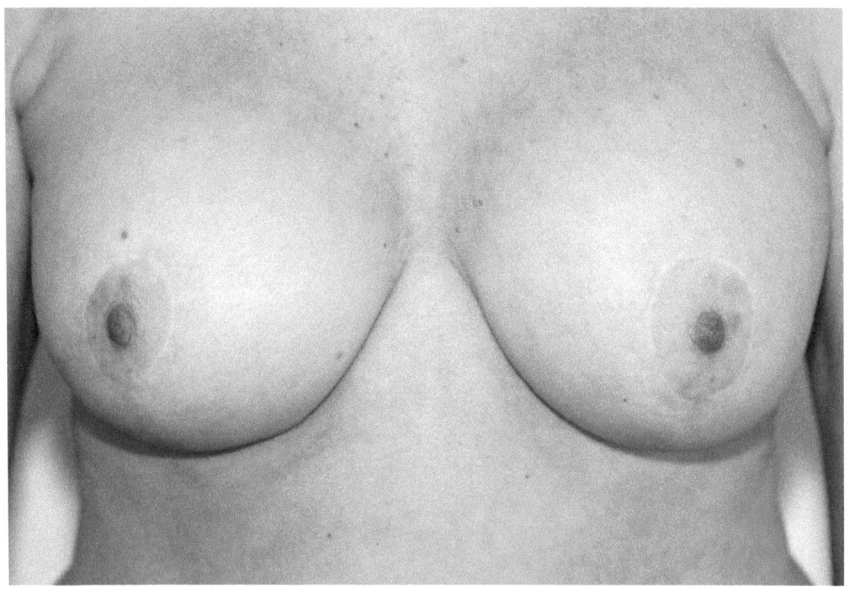

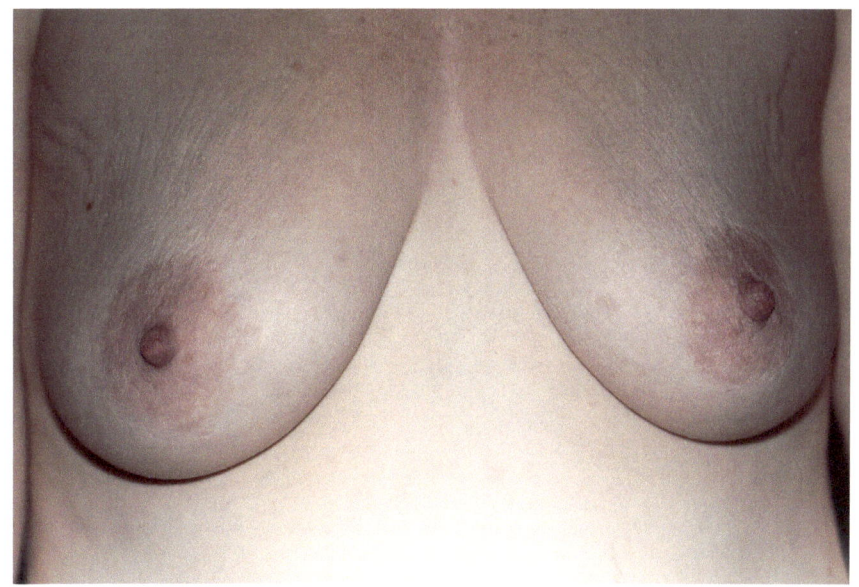

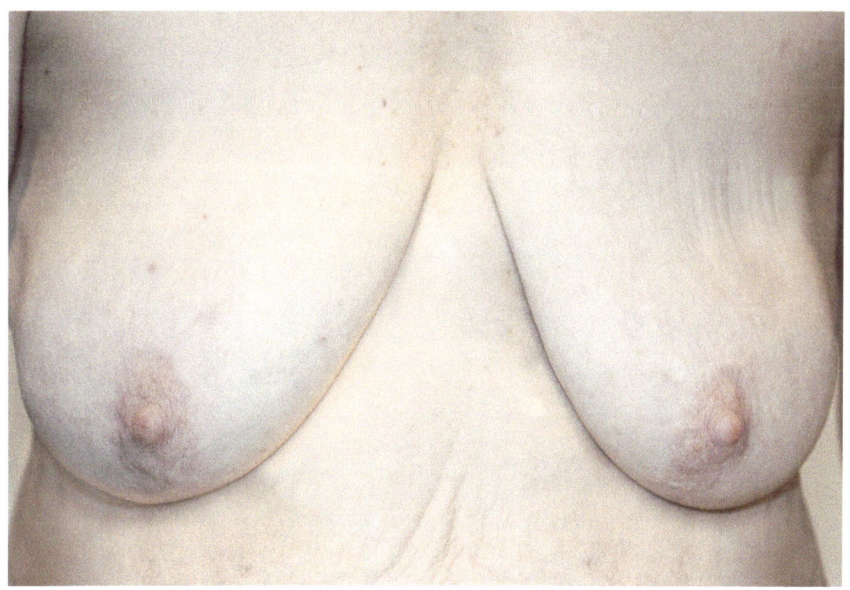

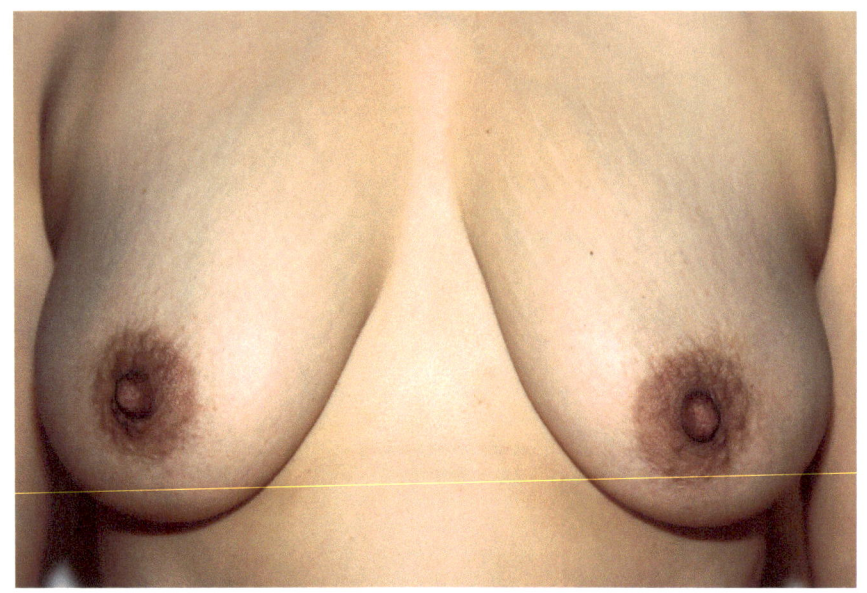

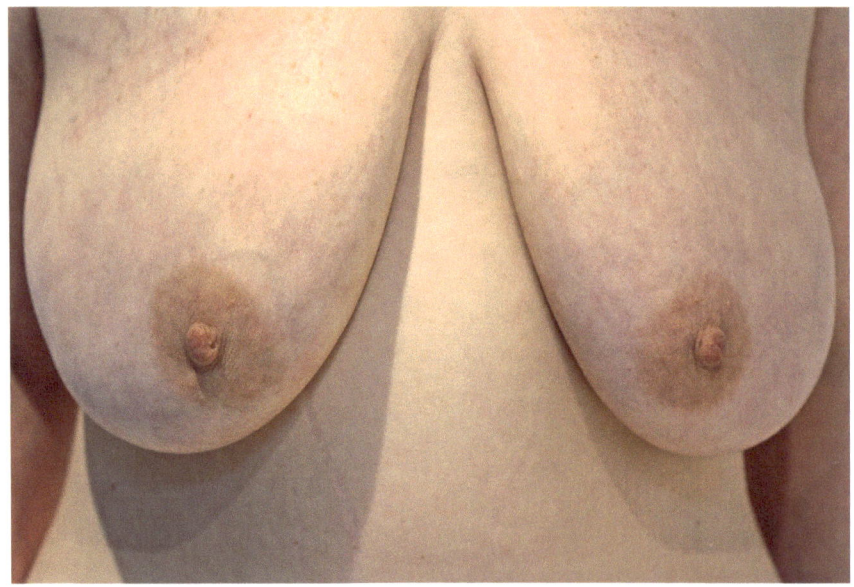

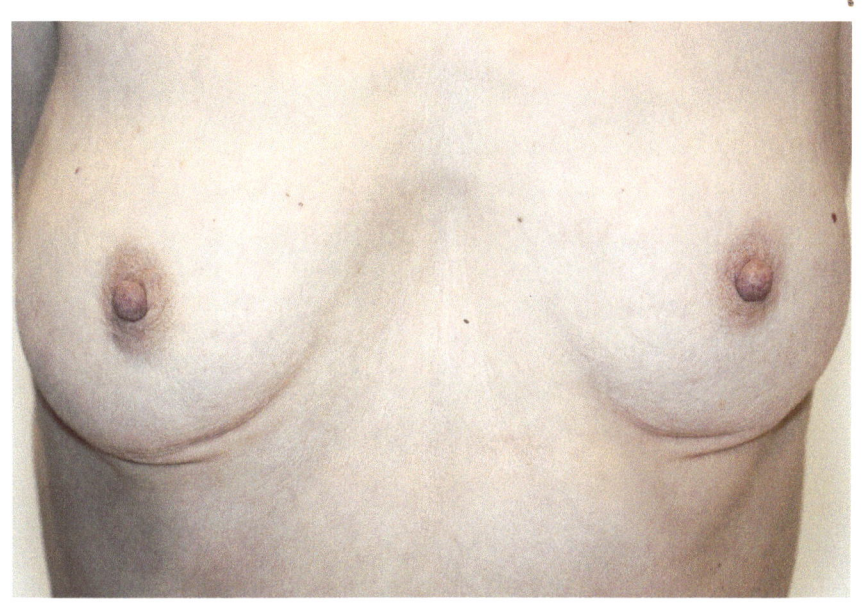

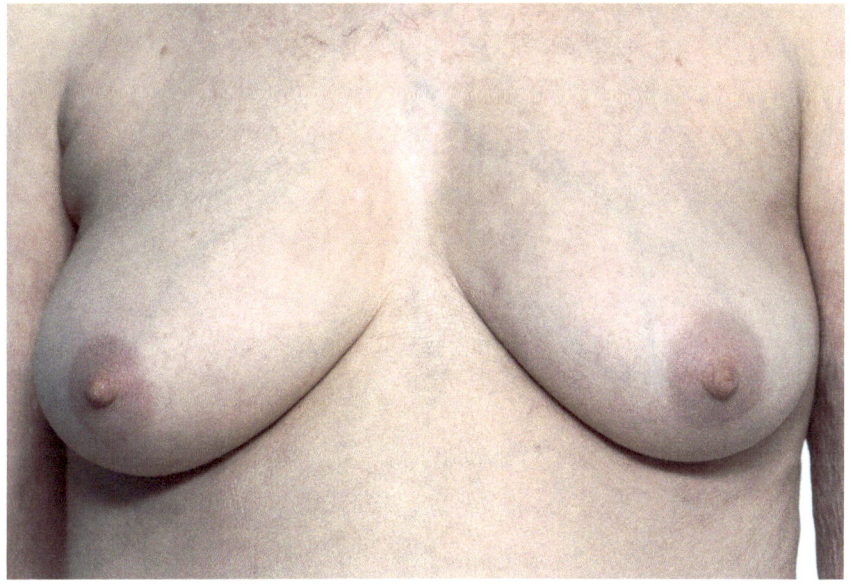

Afterword

What really matters about breasts? That is a question I posed with countless individuals. It was not a surprise to discover that attitudes regarding breasts are commensurate with one's age. Regardless of their ethnicity, education, community or socioeconomic status, people in their teens and twenties are the most conscious about the subject of breasts, and most likely have a sexualized perspective. People starting families tend to say more about the utilitarian aspects of breasts, and many still have a sexual view. By the time people are considered seniors, unless there is a health issue, the prevailing mindset about breasts is a basic lack of interest and concern.

If your breasts still have some affect on your body image and/ or sexuality you should know this: the overwhelming response by people who had an opinion about breasts was that they liked them big or small to firm or bouncy. The overall breast and nipple/areolae size, shape and color did not matter as much as the person they belonged to (and to young men, whether the respondent could see them, touch them, and/or taste them.)

So ladies, do not worry so much about your 'girls' – being healthy, loving and confident is a far bigger turn-on than any body part.

Footnotes

1. Johns Hopkins School of Medicine. "Normal Breast Development and Changes." Johns Hopkins Medicine Health Library. Web.

2. U.S. National Library of Medicine. "Gynecomastia." U.S. National Institute of Health. Web.

3. "Caring For Your Teenager." American Academy of Pediatrics, 11 May 2013. Web.

4. Industry Insights, Inc, and Scott Hackworth, CPA. International Survey on Aesthetic/Cosmetic Procedures Performed in 2013. Rep. New York City: International Society of Aesthetic Plastic Surgery–Global Statistics, 24 July 2014.

5. Rick Alteri, MD; Tracie Bertaut, APR; Durado Brooks, MD, MPH; William Chambers, PhD; Ellen Chang, ScD; Carol DeSantis, MPH; Ted Gansler, MD, MBA; Susan Gapstur, PhD; Mia Gaudet, PhD; Kerri Gober; Gery Guy, PhD, MPH; Eric Jacobs, PhD; Joan Kramer, MD; Joannie Lortet-Tieulent, MSc; Lisa A. Newman, MD, MPH; Anthony Piercy; Melissa Maitin-Shepard, MPP; Kim Miller, MPH; Ken Portier, PhD; Carolyn Runowicz, MD; Debbie Saslow, PhD; Mona Shah, MPH; Scott Simpson; Robert Smith, PhD; Kevin Stein, PhD; Lindsey Torre, MPH; Dana Wagner; Sophia Wang, PhD; Elizabeth Ward, PhD; Martin Weinstock, MD; and Joe Zou, Cancer Facts and Figures 2015. Rep. Atlanta: American Cancer Society, 2015. Print.

6. "American Cancer Society Guidelines for the Early Detection of Cancer." American Cancer Society, 29 Oct 2015. Web.

7. "Chronology of Silicon Breast Implants." PBS. Ed. WBGH Educational Foundation. PBS, n.d. Web. (Sources: The New York Times, Bloomberg Business News, AP, and American Academy of Neurology)

8. "Safety of Silicone Breast Implants" Institute of Medicine Committee on the Safety of Silicone Breast Implants; Edited by Stuart Bondurant, Virginia Ernster, and Roger Herdman. Washington (DC): National Academies Press (US); 1999.

9. United Kingdom. National Health Service; NHS Choices. How Long Do Breast Implants Last? 5 July 2014.

10. Allergan, http://www.allergan.com/assets/pdf/L3717_410_dfu.pdf, Table 7: Kaplan-Meier Risk Rates By Patient for Augmentation Cohort, Page 31, October 2014.

11. Mentor WW LLC, http://www.mentorwwllc.com Documents/01012010RevBMGWarranty.pdf, 6 October 2014.

12. Sientra, http://www.sientra.com/Content/pdfs/
The_Sientra_Limited_Warranty_and_Lifetime_Product_Replacement_Programs.pdf, 2012.

13. Nueman, William. "Mannequins Give Shape to a Venezuelan Fantasy." New
York Times Online. New York Times, 6 Nov. 2013.

14.Lynch, Patrick, 2006, Breast Anatomy normal, online illustration image.
https://commons.wikimedia.org/wiki/File:Breast_anatomy_normal.jpg

15.American Academy of Pediatrics. Breastfeeding and the Use of Human Milk. Reaffirms
Breastfeeding Guidelines 2/27/2012. Web. AAP

16.CDC National Immunization Surveys 2012 and 2013, Data, 2011 births. Web.

17. Improving Child Nutrition: The Achievable Imperative For Global Progress. UNICEF,
United Nations Publications Sales No.E.13.XX.4. April 2013. Print.

18. C. Lutter, JP Peña-Rosas, R. Perez-Escamilla. "Maternal and Child Nutrition." The
Lancet 382.9904 (n.d.): 1550-1551. Nov. 2013.

19. C. Borra, M. Iacovou, A. Sevilla. "New Evidence on Breastfeeding and Postpartum
Depression: The Importance of Understanding Women's Intentions." The Journal of
Maternal and Child Health Aug.2014. Print.

20. Dietrich, C.M., Felice, J.P., O'Sullivan, E., Rasmussen, KM. "Breastfeeding And Health
Outcomes For The Mother-Infant Dyad." Pediatric Cinics of North America, Feb.2013.

21. Carter, Shannon K., and James Mccutcheon. "Discursive Constructions of Breastfeeding
in U.S. State Laws." Women & Health 53.4

22. FourandsixTechnologies. "Photo Tampering Throughout History." Web log
post. Image Authentication and Forensics | Photo Tampering throughout History.
Fourandsix Technologies, 14 Dec. 2014. Web.

23. Hatton, Erin, and Mary Nell Trautner. "Equal Opportunity Objectification?
The Sexualization of Men and Women on the Cover of Rolling Stone." Sexuality & Culture
15.3 (2011): 256-78. Print.

www.ingramcontent.com/pod-product-compliance
Lightning Source LLC
Chambersburg PA
CBHW040827180526
45159CB00001B/90